THE LOW-CARB ATHLETE

The Official Low-Carbohydrate Nutrition Guide for Endurance and Performance

By: Ben Greenfield

www.BenGreenfieldFitness.com

Publishing services provided by Archangel Ink

ISBN: 1517371538
ISBN-13: 978-1517371531

Table of Contents

Why Choose Low Carbohydrate?

I do not recommend a "strict" low-carbohydrate diet for everyone, and I especially do not recommend it for athletes who are in training phases for which they are undergoing long hours of relatively high-intensity training (such as a professional Ironman triathlete). But there are three categories of athletes who would benefit from choosing a low-carbohydrate diet:

1) Athletes trying to lose weight.

A key component of weight loss is tapping into storage fat (adipose tissue) for energy. This fat access simply cannot happen if the body is constantly drawing on carbohydrate reserves and blood glucose for energy. In a moderate- to high-carbohydrate diet, not only does the utilization of fat for energy become far less crucial, but the body never becomes ideally efficient at using fat.

There is a growing body of evidence that a high-fat, low-carbohydrate diet causes faster and more permanent weight loss than a low-fat diet. Furthermore, appetite satiety and dietary satisfaction are significantly improved with a high-fat, low-carbohydrate diet that includes moderate protein intake. You can read about this research, as well as my own journey into becoming a fat-burning machine, at "Rewriting the Fat Burning Textbook: Part 1" and "Rewriting the Fat Burning Textbook: Part 2."

My own personal experience with a low-carbohydrate diet began with an off-season attempt to lose holiday fat pounds, followed by the stark realization that, contrary to my expectations and what I had been taught in traditional sports nutrition classes, my performance and energy levels actually improved despite a lower carbohydrate intake.

2) Athletes wanting to improve health and longevity.

When glucose is used to create energy, a high number of free radicals are produced. Free radicals are dangerous molecules that can damage normal cellular processes. The burning of fat for energy does not create this same cellular damage. In an athlete who is already creating a high number of damaging free radicals from exercise, further damage from high blood glucose levels becomes a nasty one-two combo.

In addition, the constantly elevated levels of circulating blood sugars that can be caused by a moderate- to high-carbohydrate diet are associated with nerve damage, small dense cholesterol particles (the culprits for heart disease), high morbidity, bacterial infection, cancer progression, and Alzheimer's. You can read about this damage in detail in my article "How Much Carbohydrate, Protein and Fat You Need To Stay Lean, Stay Sexy and Perform Like a Beast."

As you will learn later in this guide, simply getting your energy from non-blood-glucose-based energy sources can directly improve your quality of life and ensure that you live longer and healthier.

3) Athletes who have consistently poor performance or gastrointestinal distress while training or racing.

Because of genetic predispositions (which can actually be tested via organizations such as DNAFit), some athletes are much more sensitive to the fluctuations in blood sugar caused by carbohydrate intake. Often, the result of this sensitivity is a short-lived initial increase in energy levels after consumption of a sports bar, sports drink, gel, or other carbohydrate source, followed by a sharp and drastic drop in energy levels. But the calories from fats and proteins are utilized at a far more stable rate than carbohydrate sugar, resulting in more stable energy levels.

In addition, uncomfortable amounts of gas and bloating in athletes can be due to the high rate of bacterial activity caused by carbohydrate fermentation in the digestive tract. Many athletes experience an even greater degree of gastrointestinal distress from food allergies or intolerances to common carbohydrate sources, particularly wheat.

So who should *not* choose a low-carbohydrate diet?

First, athletes in the heat of competition, such as during an Ironman triathlon or a Spartan Beast, will certainly need a higher carbohydrate intake during the event than is recommended in this guide for the typical training week meal plan. But that's why there is also a race day plan included! In other words, even if you are eating a low-carbohydrate diet during your actual training, you will need to introduce a "slow bleed" of carbohydrates (along with some amino acids and some fats) during longer training sessions or events that bring you past the point of glycogen depletion, which is typically 60-90 minutes of moderate- to high-intensity exercise or 90 minutes to 2 hours of low- to moderate-intensity exercise. I discuss the reasons for this in detail in the podcast episode "Five Simple Steps To Turning Yourself Into a Fat Burning Machine."

Next, athletes going through an extremely heavy block of training *that is a higher load than they are accustomed to,* such as a triathlon camp that involves 25-40 hours of training per week, will also need a higher carbohydrate intake (although this volume of training combined with higher carbohydrate intake is not healthy, it is a necessary sacrifice for injecting large doses of endurance into the body).

Finally, individuals with diseases or conditions that disable the ability to properly metabolize fats and proteins (such as gallbladder removal) may also need to eat a higher percentage of daily calories from carbohydrates, since they simply cannot digest fats very well. Some of this can be managed with digestive enzymes that can assist with fat digestion, but ultimately, some folks simply can't handle extremely high amounts of fat combined with low amounts of carbohydrate. You might think that simply adding in more protein would be the answer, but then you begin to play with issues related to protein toxicity.

Answering Objections

Once your training partners, family, or other friends learn that you're eating fewer carbohydrates, you're guaranteed to hear several objections and see some raised eyebrows. Typically, the criticism of a low-carbohydrate diet falls into three categories of questions:

Objection #1: *Isn't glucose and carbohydrate necessary for energy during exercise?*

As mentioned earlier in this guide, directly burning blood glucose for fuel causes a significant amount of free radical damage compared to burning storage carbohydrate, storage fats, or circulating fats in the bloodstream. This type of fuel utilization occurs in the endurance athlete trained to eat a gel every 20 minutes during every single training session, or to constantly have a sports drink on the edge of the pool and a bowl of pasta waiting at home to refuel after the workout.

While cells can certainly burn glucose for energy, fat is a preferred energy source in nearly every cell, and especially for the mitochondria, which are the energy-creating organelles within most cells. Until extremely high exercise intensities are achieved (rarely the case among endurance athletes) or until the human body has exercised for two to three hours continuously, fat is completely useable as an energy source. Specifically, natural saturated fats, omega-3 fatty acids, and medium chain triglycerides are extremely dense energy sources that produce very few damaging byproducts from their metabolic use for energy.

The specific parts of the body that do need glucose on a daily basis are the brain, the nerves, special proteins called "glycoproteins" (which form compounds such as mucus), and cells within the immune system, the gastrointestinal tract, and the kidneys. But the total daily amount of glucose calories required by these parts of the body is about 500-700 carbohydrate calories, and not the 1500-2000 carbohydrate calories consumed by most endurance athletes!

Objection #2: *Isn't fat dangerous for cholesterol-related heart disease, as well as posing an increased risk of weight gain?*

No. Not only does a high-fat, low-carbohydrate diet perform better for weight loss compared to a low-fat, high-carbohydrate diet, but there is no evidence that the cholesterol particles derived from fat increase the risk of heart disease–unless fat consumption is paired with a moderate to high intake of starchy, sugary carbohydrate sources. It is at that point that cholesterol can become oxidized and lead to risk of heart disease.

The entire idea that high cholesterol causes heart disease is a flawed hypothesis, and entire books have been written on it. A very good place to start your journey into learning about the positive and healthy properties of fats would be the website www.cholesterol-and-health.com (which is in no manner affiliated with this guide–it is simply a helpful resource).

Objection #3: *Don't you need to load with carbohydrate before a race?*

Once you begin eating a low-carbohydrate diet, your body will, within two weeks, become more efficient at burning fat (although it's important to realize that it takes up to six months before you really start to "feel good" during workouts, and one to two years before you are fully fat adapted). This means that you will need relatively fewer carbohydrates during race week or the day before a race, since your body develops an enhanced ability to conserve storage carbohydrate (glycogen) and also an increased ability to utilize fat as a fuel, both during rest and on race day.

What this means is that an entire week of traditional carbohydrate loading and high sugar intake will not be necessary, and if your goal is weight loss, health, or longevity, it may actually end up doing more harm than good. Since I have shifted to a lower carbohydrate intake, I have found that the 85-90% carbohydrate diet I was eating during race week is no longer necessary. The primary changes I now make during race week are A) a carbohydrate-dense breakfast the day before and the morning of the race; and B) more frequent snacking in the last several days leading up to the race (not allowing a feeling of hunger to set in); C) a few extra carbohydrates with dinner (such as 200-300 calories of extra carbs) from a source such as sweet potatoes, yams, or white rice. Sure, this would still be considered "carbohydrate loading," but not in the common tradition of loading, which typically includes 7-10 days of high carbohydrate intake before an event, with a gradual increase of carbs up to 90% carb intake the day before a race!

Low-Carbohydrate Diet Overview

The average athlete, based on current recommendations by most personal trainers, coaches, sports nutritionists, books, magazines, etc. eats a diet of about 50-60%+ carbohydrate, 20-30% protein, and 20-30% fat. The major problem with this type of dietary intake is not primarily the percentages of carbs, proteins, and fats (unless you are indeed trying to eat a low-carbohydrate diet), but instead the source from which many of these foods are commonly derived—cookies, crackers, pasta, biscotti, scones, bagels, muffins, energy bars, juice, processed trail mixes, etc. Each of these foods and others like them are very high in vegetable oils, inflammatory omega-6 fatty acids, preservatives, processed ingredients, potential food allergens, refined sugars and, perhaps most annoyingly to the majority of athletes, highly fermentable carbohydrates that cause gas, bloating, and constipation.

The low-carbohydrate diet for athletes that you're going to find in this book addresses all these issues, and includes the following components:

Higher Fat Percentage: With a macronutrient percentage of closer to *50-60% fat, 20-30% carbohydrate, and 20-30% protein,* the low-carbohydrate diet not only naturally eliminates many of the unhealthy food ingredients present in a higher-carbohydrate diet, but also introduces more stable energy levels, less inflammation, and better weight loss. While very low carbohydrate percentages that you'd find on a strict ketogenic diet (5-10% carbs) will not sustain heavy bouts of high-intensity exercise or voluminous training, the slightly higher percentage of carbohydrates you'll find in this diet are perfect for lasting health, longevity, weight loss, or elimination of digestive issues from food intolerances.

Yes, you read right. The percentages listed above are not what you'll find in a strict "ketogenic" diet. Strict ketogenesis can be difficult and uncomfortable for most and is not extremely practical from a social eating perspective, either. For a ketogenic diet, you'd be closer to 80-85% fat, 10-15% protein, and 5-10% carbohydrate. However, by saving the majority of your day's carbohydrate intake for the end of the day, and preferably consuming them in a post-exercise scenario anywhere from one to three hours after your workout, you will indeed be in a state of ketosis the entire day leading up to that carbohydrate "feeding." Many nutritionists refer to this practice as "cyclic ketosis" or a "cycling low-carb diet."

Carbohydrate Cycling: If long-term carbohydrate deprivation and depletion of storage carbohydrate levels are accompanied by frequent bouts of training, then your immune system can eventually become depressed, physical performance and mood can decline, and risk of overtraining can increase. For this reason, storage carbohydrate should be "reloaded" once per week, preferably on a higher-volume training day during which the increased carbohydrate intake will be less damaging to the body. This is a practice that can be combined with the "cyclic low-carb" approach described earlier. The meal plan you'll find in this guide is a six-day, low-carbohydrate diet with one day of moderate to high carbohydrate intake, and that higher-carbohydrate-intake day should preferably be the hardest training day of the week (which is typically a Saturday or Sunday for most athletes). *It's very important to note that if you aren't the type of exerciser or athlete who has a very high-volume training day of the week, this extra carbohydrate "refeed" day will probably not be necessary for you, especially if you're already doing the cyclic low-carb approach with miniature carb refeeds at the end of each day. But if you really find yourself frequently "running into the wall," you'll definitely want to include this day.*

Fasted Sessions: If your goal is weight loss, then more-rapid fat burning results can be attained by including fasted morning exercise sessions in your program. To implement these, simply wake up in the morning and engage in 20-60 minutes of exercise before eating anything (coffee is fine). It is preferable that the exercise be an easy aerobic session, since hard training sessions are more difficult to do on an empty stomach and may result in "junk" training, overtraining, or simply too much stress early in the day. Usually, an easy swim, easy bike ride, yoga session, or even a walk with the dog is sufficient (and the more sunshine, the better, as it helps to jumpstart your circadian rhythm and normalize your sleep patterns). Ideally, this session should be done at some point during a twelve-hour fast (e.g., you stop eating at 8pm the night before, then wake up and get your easy exercise session in at 7am, then eat breakfast anytime at 8am or after). If exercising in a fasted state in the morning is not possible for you, then it would be preferable to include a longer fasted session, in which dinner is completed 3-4 hours prior to bedtime, and then breakfast is eaten 1-2 hours after waking, which, with 7-8 hours of sleep, can result in a 12+ hour fast. You do not need to include fasted workout sessions or fasts every day of the week, but you absolutely can, and there's no risk of "starvation mode" or metabolic damage as long as you're actually eating sufficient calories the rest of the day. I personally include these sessions six to seven times per week. Finally, for athletes, this morning exercise session will probably not be your "main" training session of the day. Your main, hard, intense or voluminous training should actually be later in the day, before dinner, when your post-workout protein synthesis, body temperature, and reaction time peaks, and before a meal when you'll ideally be eating the majority of your day's carbohydrates.

Carbohydrate Intake During Long Workouts: This is where things get interesting because there are two options:

Option 1: Some people like to "train low, race high" with respect to carbohydrates. This is what I personally did for several years. It means I trained with a low-carbohydrate diet most of the time but used a large number of carbohydrates during the actual race.

If you use this approach, your gut needs to be trained to absorb as many calories as it will be taking in on race day. So if you are, say, a Half-Ironman or Ironman endurance athlete, about once every two weeks, one of your long workouts (typically the bike or run) will need to be accompanied by the use of gels, sports drinks, bars, or other carbohydrate sources that you plan on using during the race. This is basically "training your gut." You don't need to do this very frequently, but just enough to allow you to become used to the nutrition plan you will be implementing during race day. Although volume will vary significantly depending on one's size and training status, calorie intake for these carbohydrate-fueled long workouts for males will be 300-450 calories per hour on the bike and 200-300 calories per hour on the run, and for females will be 250-400 calories per hour on the bike and 150-250 calories per hour on the run. All your other long workouts can be minimally fueled, with a half to a quarter as many calories as you plan on consuming on race day, and you do not need to fuel at all during any workouts that are an hour or less. This practice of "minimally" training your gut to digest higher amounts of carbohydrates will help you to become fat adapted, and is much different than the typical practice that athletes implement of fueling every training session as though it were a race.

Option 2: Train low, race low. This approach involves minimum carbohydrate utilization during training (similar to option 1) but also includes minimal carbohydrate utilization during the actual event. The advantage is that this is a good solution if you're eating low carb for health reasons, or you have lots of difficulty with "energy highs and lows" from typical sports gels and drinks, or you have lots of stomach distress from all those fermentable simple carbohydrates in typical sports gels and drinks, or you want all the cognitive enhancement, focus, and superior long-term energy that can come from competing in a state of "ketosis."

The disadvantage is that it can be hard to push yourself really hard if you're not taking in many carbohydrates during an event that is both voluminous and intense, and for someone who is, for example, attempting to do a Half Ironman in five hours or less or an Ironman in ten hours or less, the intensity is high enough so that "racing low carbohydrate" may not be realistic. You would actually have to experiment during longer race simulation training sessions to see if this approach works for you. What I've found is that if you cut your "normal" carb intake in half (e.g., cut from 400 calories of carbs/hr down to, say, 200 calories of carbs/hr), then fill in those calorie "holes" with A) about 10g of amino acids per hour and B) 50–100 calories of MCT or coconut oil per hour, then you can generally sustain long, intense efforts just fine. But you must, must, must try this in your training before you do it in a race.

However, if you're staying purely aerobic during your race and not "redlining," then a low- to no-carb approach can work. It's simple, really. Here's what you do:

Thirty to sixty minutes prior to the race: 1g sodium (i.e., a chicken bouillon cube—this keeps your blood pressure high enough on a low carb intake), 5-10g BCAAs or EAAs (branched chain amino acids or essential amino acids—and the latter are far more complete and superior) and 2-3 tablespoons medium chain triglyceride oil or coconut oil.

Every hour during event: 5-10g amino acids (e.g., the EAA's mentioned above) and 100-150 calories of a slow-release starch such as UCAN SuperStarch per hour. Also (optional, and discussed more in the supplementary chapter at the end of this book), is the product "VESPA," a unique wasp-based amino acid product that allows you to tap into your own fat as a fuel more readily. If you find that UCAN "ferments" or doesn't sit well with you, a couple other products I like are "Infinit-E" by Millennium Sports (use 50% discount code MSTBG09) and "ISKIATE Endurance" by Natural Force (use 10% code BEN10)

Basic Food Overview: Since you'll be eating a high percentage of fats, your kitchen will be stocked with full-fat coconut milk, coconut oil, coconut shavings, avocados, olives, extra virgin olive oil, macadamia nuts, pumpkin seeds, walnuts, sardines, salmon, cheese, heavy cream, whole fat yogurt, and fatty cuts of beef. For added protein, you'll also have eggs and chicken. Carbohydrate sources will be clean-burning, easily digested fuels, including sweet potato, yam, white rice, quinoa, amaranth, millet, and fruit. Liberal consumption of non-starchy vegetables is also included. For a whole list of other healthy pantry foods to have around for your diet, read this helpful article about my own pantry: (http://bit.ly/1PaQu4S).

Supplements: Your supplementation protocol is going to widely vary, and although the best supplementation protocol should be based on blood testing that identifies your specific needs and deficiencies, you should at least include three basic foundation supplements that are highly beneficial for health and performance in the absence of a moderate to high carbohydrate intake: a high-quality multivitamin, a daily electrolyte supplement and an omega-3 fatty acid source such as fish oil or spirulina (for the latter, I like a product called "EnergyBits," an organic, vegan-friendly spirulina source—use 10% discount code BEN here). For added digestive support when switching to high fat intake, you may want to include a digestive enzyme prior to your higher fat meals. Then, for added performance and recovery (again, not necessary, but an option if you want "better living through science"), you can include a workout and injury recovery supplement that contains natural anti-inflammatories and some kind of adaptogenic herb complex to assist with hormonal balance. I realize that I've really skimmed over many of these items, but there is more on supplementation in the chapter on supplements at the end of this book.

The next several pages will introduce you to grocery shopping, then your meal plan for a regular week of training, a fueling plan for long workouts, a race week meal plan, and a race day meal plan.

Please be warned that as you make the transition to a low-carbohydrate diet, you will go through a period of "ketoadaptation," during which your body becomes accustomed to burning fatty acids as a primary fuel. Depending on how high your carbohydrate intake was prior to embarking upon this low-carbohydrate dietary approach, you will go through a period of low energy, fatigue, grumpiness, and subpar workout performance that will last for anywhere from four days to two weeks.

This drop in energy is completely normal and will subside after at least two weeks. Consider yourself warned, and as you have probably guessed, you should not switch to this diet if you are two weeks or less away from an important race or competition.

Many people find that drinking more good, clean water, along with adding a few extra servings of electrolytes, trace minerals and sea salt per day can help tremendously with this low energy, since part of the feeling of dizziness and malaise can be due to a drop in blood pressure as your body sheds carbohydrates and water.

Grocery Shopping List

For many of the pantry-based and packaged items, I'd highly recommend you use a service called "Thrive Market," which is like Amazon mixed with Whole Foods!

Carbohydrate Sources:

- Sweet potato and/or yam (these are considered starchy vegetables)
- White rice, wild rice, and/or quinoa
- Gluten-free bread or wrap
- Organic fruit (you can choose your favorites, but good ones are raspberries, papaya, banana, strawberries, peaches)
- Organic vegetables:
  - Cabbage
  - Butter lettuce leaves
  - Spinach
  - Kale, bok choy, and/or Swiss chard
  - Broccoli
  - Cauliflower
  - Brussels sprouts
  - Bell peppers
  - Nori (seaweed)

- Sauerkraut
- Garlic
- Cucumber
- Crimini mushrooms
- Red onions
- Green onions
- Parsley
- Zucchini
- Shallots
- Sugar snap peas
- Cilantro
- Bean sprouts

Protein Sources:

- Wild Atlantic salmon
- Sardines
- Herring
- Anchovies
- Cod
- Shrimp
- Organic grass-fed beef (choose fattier cuts)
- Organic free-range chicken
- Omega-3 enriched eggs from free-range chickens
- Some kind of organic organ meat (I prefer liver from USWellnessMeats)

Fat Sources (in addition to proteins listed on the previous page):

- Macadamia nuts
- Brazil nuts
- Almonds
- Pumpkin seeds
- Walnuts
- Hemp seeds
- Sesame seeds
- Chia seeds
- Avocados
- Olives
- Coconut oil
- Whole full-fat coconut milk
- Unsweetened coconut shavings
- Whole Greek yogurt
- Feta or goat cheese

Beverages:

- Coconut water kefir
- Kombucha
- Teeccino
- Mineral-rich sparkling water such as San Pellegrino, Perrier, or Gerolsteiner
- Bone Broth

Condiments:

- Ghee (clarified butter) if you can get it at the grocery store
- Lemon juice
- Extra virgin olive oil
- Apple cider vinegar
- Rice vinegar
- Sesame oil
- Non-soy soy sauce alternative (such as coconut aminos)
- Minced garlic
- Capers
- Lemon
- Water chestnuts
- Ginger
- Cayenne pepper
- Fish sauce
- Wasabi

Additional Recommendations:

LivingFuel SuperGreens Meal Replacement. If you must get quick nutrition and don't have time to cook, two to three heaping scoops of the Living Fuel SuperGreens mixed in ½ cup full-fat coconut milk or water can be used as a meal replacement for ANY of the meals on this plan. For an even lower carbohydrate option, such as when you are sitting at the office or late at night, the same substitution can be made, but with Living Fuel SuperProtein.

Meal Plan for Regular Training Days

This is the meal plan that you will stick to for six days of each week (remember that there is still one day per week that will involve a higher carbohydrate intake). For each meal, choose one option. If you are a male or a large person, choose the higher range of caloric volume (i.e., if it says two to three eggs, eat three, or if it says one medium-large sweet potato, choose large).

Breakfast (choose 1):

Whenever possible, complete any of your easy workouts in the morning before breakfast. For added benefit, do not eat within two hours of bedtime.

- Eggs: 2–3 eggs. Scramble eggs in coconut oil or ghee with mix of your choice of vegetables, and serve with sea salt, black pepper, and 1 fried or baked sweet potato, yam, or taro. Serve with a liberal amount of steamed vegetables of choice, and top with feta or goat cheese or full-fat yogurt.
- ¾–1 cup whole full-fat coconut milk blended with ice, cinnamon, 1 tablespoon nut butter, 1 tablespoon coconut oil, and 1 handful nuts of choice.
- 2-3 scoops Living Fuel Supergreens or LivingProtein with 3 tablespoons chia seeds or 1 handful macadamia nuts or Brazil nuts.

- ¾–1 cup whole Greek yogurt with 1 handful macadamia nuts and 2 tablespoons chia seeds.

- Keto tea (turmeric tea—am a fan of this recipe (http://bit.ly/1y7YUTv) or you can simply buy Tumi turmeric bags) or Bulletproof Coffee (all coffee details/recipe here: http://bit.ly/1A0xfWa)
- This High Fat Smoothie: (youtube.com/watch?v=x0cSlmwsFwY)

Snack 1:

- No mid-morning snack necessary on any day except the hardest workout day of the week, in which case you'll be using the next meal plan (don't worry, infrequent eating doesn't cause your metabolism to drop). If you get extremely hungry between breakfast and lunch, have a couple tablespoons of coconut oil, or better yet, simply some sparkling water with gum. In your first couple weeks adapting to this diet, you may also want to add in electrolyte tablets, electrolyte capsules, or sea salt with your water.

Lunch:

- Large vegetable salad. You can chop and serve as many non-starchy vegetables as you'd like, salt and pepper to taste, and drench in 3-4 tablespoons extra virgin olive oil or macadamia nut oil, and apple cider vinegar. Include 2 handfuls black olives, 1–2 handfuls pumpkin seeds, and ½–1 sliced avocado. A quality, organic cheese or full-fat yogurt can also be added for extra calories.

- Alternatively, you can have leftovers from the previous night's dinner, which you'll end up doing quite often.

- A cup of hot or cold bone broth with lunch is also fine, and I actually encourage it. You can learn everything you need to know about bone broth here: (bonebroth.com/?ref=17).

Dinner: (Choose 1)

- 2–3 eggs and ½–1 avocado, chopped and sautéed in coconut oil and wrapped in kale, bok choy, Swiss chard, or cabbage leaf. Salt and pepper to taste. (Do not eat this if you had eggs for breakfast already.) Alternatively, instead of using eggs + avocado, you can use 6–9 oz of herring or anchovies to fill wrap. Serve with a cooked white rice, wild rice and/or quinoa, mashed sweet potato, yam, or taro. For a starch substitute, you can also do sweet potato fries.
- 6–9oz salted beef or salmon. Rub with minced garlic and serve with lemon juice and as many non-starchy vegetables as you'd like, steamed or sautéed, and lightly salted. Season with salt, pepper, kelp, kombu, and/or dulse seasoning. Serve with a ¾–1 cup of cooked white rice, wild rice, and/or quinoa, mashed sweet potato, yam, or taro.
- 6–9oz chicken. Prepare as desired and serve with ½–1 avocado and as many non-starchy vegetables as you'd like, steamed or sautéed, and lightly salted. Season with salt, pepper, kelp, kombu, and/or dulse seasoning. Serve with a ¾–1 cup of cooked white rice, wild rice, and/or quinoa, mashed sweet potato, yam, or taro.
- ***Spicy Shrimp & Onions***. Use 6–9 large shrimp and serve with a ¾–1 cup of cooked white rice, wild rice and/or quinoa, mashed sweet potato, yam, or taro.
- ***Chicken Skewers with Almond Sauce***. This is a more family style recipe, so volume will depend on the number of people you're feeding, but you should eat the equivalent of two small-medium breasts, with 1–2

tablespoons of the almond sauce. Cut chicken breasts in ½ thickness strips. Marinate in non-soy soy sauce alternative for about two hours. BBQ chicken on skewer or bake at 350 until cooked through. Plate on a big bed of spinach.

Almond Sauce:

- ¼ cup creamy almond butter
- 2 tsp raw honey
- 2 tsp gluten-free soy sauce alternative such as coconut aminos
- 1 Tbsp rice vinegar
- 2 tsp grated ginger
- ½ cup full-fat coconut milk

- Combine all ingredients in a saucepan over medium heat. Cook until it thickens, about 5 min.

- ***Cod Dish***
  - 1 tsp extra virgin olive oil or macadamia oil or avocado oil
  - 2 cod fillets (you can multiply this recipe by the number of people you're feeding, but you eat the equivalent of 1 medium-large fillet)
  - 2 Tbsp unsalted butter or ghee or coconut oil
  - 3 Tbsp salted capers
  - a handful of fresh parsley, finely chopped
  - one lemon

Drizzle olive oil or macadamia oil onto the fish fillets and season with salt and pepper. Gently heat a non-stick frying pan, add the fish, skin down, and cook until the skin starts to color and turn golden and crisp. Turn up the heat slightly and add the fresh butter; after a couple of minutes, turn the fish over. Finish cooking until the butter begins to turn brown (be careful not to let it go black). Add the capers and chopped parsley and finish with a good squeeze of lemon juice to deglaze the pan. Remove the fish from the pan and serve immediately.*Serve with roasted veggies/potatoes:*

- 3 sweet potatoes, halved
- 1 bell pepper, cut in ½- in cubes
- 1 onion, quartered
- 1 zucchini, cubed
- ¼ cup balsamic vinegar
- 2 Tbsp olive oil
- 1 tsp salt
- Black pepper

Before roasting, boil potatoes for 20 min. or until potatoes can easily be pierced with a fork. Eat the equivalent of ¾–1 cup of this.

- ***Miracle Noodles with Chicken***. (This is just one example of a good Miracle Noodles recipe—more on their website. To read why I'm a big fan of these, go here: (http://bit.ly/1Nsch9y).

Cook 150-250 calories worth of Miracle Noodles according to package directions. Meanwhile, sauté sliced chicken breast in 1 teaspoon olive oil with red bell pepper, half of a chopped cucumber, a handful of sliced red onions, a handful of sliced mushrooms, a handful of chopped broccoli, a handful of spinach, and one crushed garlic clove. Serve over Miracle Noodles. This meal is slightly lower calorie and would be best for a completely easy or recovery day.

- ***Thai Cucumber Salad and Tom Kha Gai***
  - 1 English cucumber OR 2 field cucumbers (if using organic, leave the skin on; otherwise, wash well or peel it off)
  - 1 shallot, minced (OR substitute ¼ cup minced purple onion)
  - 2 green (spring) onions, finely sliced

- 1 fresh red chili, deseeded and minced fine, OR ¼ cup diced red bell pepper
- ½ cup fresh coriander/cilantro, roughly chopped
- ¼ cup ground or roughly chopped nuts of choice (not peanuts)

Dressing:

- 2 Tbsp fish sauce
- juice of ½ lime
- 1–2 cloves garlic, minced
- ½ tsp shrimp paste (available by the jar at Asian stores)
- 1 Tbsp non-soy soy sauce alternative
- ¼ to ½ tsp cayenne pepper (to taste)
- 1 to 1 ½ tsp coconut sugar

Cut the cucumber in half lengthwise, then repeat with each half until you have a number of long strips. Now slice the other way to create bite-size rectangular chunks. Place in a salad bowl.

Add the shallot, green onion, chili/red pepper, and coriander to the salad bowl (keep back a little extra coriander for a garnish).

Combine the dressing ingredients together in a cup, stirring to dissolve the shrimp paste. Taste-test it for sweet-sour balance, adding more sugar if it's too sour for your taste.

Pour dressing over the salad and toss well.

Top with the ground/chopped nuts, plus extra coriander. If desired, garnish with a slice of lime. Serve immediately, or cover and refrigerate for up to 3 hours.

- ***Tom Kha Gai***
  - 1 quart chicken broth
  - 1 can of full-fat coconut milk
  - ¼ tsp dried chili flakes
  - 1 tsp freshly grated ginger
  - juice of 1 lemon
  - sea salt (to taste)
  - 2 cups cubed cooked chicken (optional)
  - 2 green onions, chopped (optional)
  - chopped cilantro (optional)

Bring the stock to a boil, skim any foam that rises to the top, and add full-fat coconut milk, lemon juice, chili flakes, ginger, and optional chicken. Simmer for about 15 minutes. Season to taste with salt. Ladle into soup bowls or mugs and garnish with cilantro and green onions.

One serving is a medium-large bowl of soup and 1–2 cups of salad.

- ***Shrimp Sushi Salad***

Marinated Shrimp:

  - 12 shrimp peeled and deveined (may need to add more depending on number of people you're feeding)
  - 5 Tbsp sesame oil
  - 5 Tbsp soy sauce alternative
  - 2 Tbsp rice vinegar
  - 1 clove garlic
  - ½ red chili
  - 2 tsp fresh ginger, peeled and minced

Making the marinade:

- Mix the ingredients for the marinade in a bowl and add the shrimp. Make sure the marinade covers all of the shrimp. Put in the fridge for 4–8 hours. Place the shrimp on a baking sheet and broil. This should take no longer than 2–5 min. Shrimp turns pink when it is done. Cook the leftover marinade from the shrimp on medium heat until it boils. Then let it cool and use it as the dressing.
- Cook 1 cup of white rice, wild rice, and/or quinoa.

Add:

- 2 Tbsp rice vinegar
- 1 tsp sesame oil

Salad

- Marinated and cooked shrimp
- White rice, wild rice, and/or quinoa
- 1 large broccoli stalk, broken into 1-inch pieces
- 1 green onion
- 2 avocados, cut into cubes
- 12 mushrooms (shiitake or whatever you prefer), cut in quarters
- 1 handful sugar snap peas, cut in half
- 1 handful bean sprouts
- ½ cucumber, cut into sticks
- 8 sheets nori seaweed, cut into 2×2-inch squares
- 1 handful roasted sesame seeds
- 1 handful cilantro

Blanch the broccoli (pour boiled water over it, let it set for two minutes, then throw it in ice-cold water). Divide the rice into large bowls and top it with all the vegetables mixed together. Drizzle the rest of the marinade over the salad, top it with sesame seeds and cilantro, and serve it with wasabi and soy sauce alternative. One serving is the equivalent of a medium to large bowl with 5–6 shrimp on it.

Pre or Post-Workout Snack:

(choose just one—only necessary before or after workouts of 1+ hour in duration or on high-volume exercise days)

- ***Bar***

My preferred brands include ingredients like organic chia seeds, organic raw almond butter, organic agave syrup, non-GMO rice protein, organic cocoa and organic chocolate liquor, etc. Good brands are Hammer Recovery Bar or Hammer Vegan Recovery Bar (use 15% discount code 80244 here: (hammernutrition.com), LaraBar, Nogii Bar, Quest Bar, Zing Bar, or HeathWarrior Bar.

- ***Chia Slurry***

Set 3–4 tablespoon of chia seeds in a small bowl of water and place in the refrigerator for 2–24 hours (the longer they're soaking the more chia goodness will get absorbed from them).

Add lemon juice and stevia to taste, and voila! Eat like jello.

- ***Pemmican or Jerky***

Eat "tube" of organic, pastured pemmican from US Wellness Meats. Alternatively, you can eat 200-300 calories of all-natural jerky from US Wellness Meats. The Warrior bars from Onnit are also quite good.

- ***LivingFuel***

Combine:

- 1–2 large scoops of Living Fuel Supergreens or Superberry with
- 2–4 ounces full-fat, organic, BPA-free coconut milk

- 1 Tbsp almond butter
- 1 tsp cinnamon
- a handful of coconut flakes (unsweetened)
- a Tbsp of chia seeds.

You can blend this, shake it in a mixer bottle, or simply stir it all together with a spoon.

- ***Coconut milk with protein powder***

Mix one scoop protein powder into 3–4oz full-fat coconut milk, stir or blend and eat.

- **1-2 cups bone broth.** You can drink this hot or cold.

Snack 3:

(choose one—only necessary during workouts of 2+ hours in duration—you can also refer to "long workout fueling" section towards end of this book)

- Into water bottle during workouts: 3–4 tablespoons chia seeds or 1 tablespoon MCT oil, 1 tablespoon raw honey, 1 tablespoon electrolytes or sea salts, 5–10 grams amino acids. You can find plenty of suggestions/resources for electrolytes and amino acids at here: (greenfieldfitnesssystems.com)
- 5–10g amino acids 30 minutes prior to and during your main workouts. Use BCAAs or EAAs (branched chain amino acids or essential amino acids—and the latter are far more complete and superior).
- During long workouts, a combination of Athlytes (you can also get those from Millennium Sports with 50% discount code MSTBG09) at 2 every 30 minutes + a fat-based energy gel of your choosing at 100-150 calories every 30 minutes + 5–10g amino acids every 60 minutes.
- Natural Force ISKIATE Endurance—1–2 servings per hour. You can get 10% discount with code BEN10 at

NaturalForce website:
(mynaturalforce.com/#bengreenfield)

Drinks:

- Acceptable drinks include teas, mushroom teas, soda water, coconut kefir, Zevia soda, any soda water or regular water with additions such as stevia, essential oils, lemon juice, etc. Look for beverages that have 20 calories or less.
- As far as alcohol, if you would like, as a substitute for any of the post-workout snacks, you can include a glass of red wine with 10g of amino acids.

Meal Plan for the Biggest Training Day of the Week (Carb Refeed Day)

This is the meal plan that you will eat for just one day of the week, preferably your biggest, hardest day of training (for most, this falls on a weekend). While this isn't a full-on "cheat day," it certainly includes a higher caloric intake and less "clean eating" than the other days of the week. This is called a carb refeed day.

You will not see any nutritional supplements on this meal plan, but you can continue to take the supplements you were taking the other six days of the week.

Breakfast (choose 1):

- ***Waffles or Pancakes***

1. Begin by sprouting and fermenting millet, quinoa, oats, or buckwheat.
2. Wash them with water four or five time and leave to soak them in filtered water overnight in a glass bowl with a plate on top.
3. In the morning, wash and rinse your grains thoroughly and cover with filtered water again. This time, add about 1 T of whey or the juice of half a lemon to the water and cover again for 12–24 hours.

4. Rinse the grains and strain out the water. They are now ready to use.

For your recipe, take

- 3 cups of your sprouted, fermented grain
- 4 organic pastured eggs
- 3 –4 Tbsp grass-fed butter or coconut oil
- 2 tsp baking soda
- 1 Tbsp vanilla

Blend all ingredients in the food processor for at least 5 minutes until nice and smooth. Use in your favorite waffle iron. This batter works for pancakes as well. Serve with grass-fed butter or almond butter, a dollop of organic, grass-fed yogurt or kefir, and a small amount of sliced bananas or berries of your choice.

- ***Hot Power Quinoa***

To sprout and ferment your quinoa:

1. Wash it with water four or five time and leave to soak in filtered water over night in a glass bowl with a plate on top.
2. In the morning, wash and rinse thoroughly and cover with filtered water again. This time add about 1 T of whey or the juice of half a lemon to the water and cover again for 12–24 hours.
3. Rinse the quinoa and strain out the water. It is now ready to use.
4. Cook a serving of quinoa for 20 minutes over medium heat on stovetop, and then remove from heat and stir in 1 tablespoon of almond butter, a pinch of sea salt, a tablespoon of chia seeds or unsweetened coconut flakes, 1/2 teaspoon vanilla and 1 teaspoon cinnamon.

- Egg, avocado, and tomato breakfast sandwich—Use two slices of gluten-free bread or a gluten-free wrap and eat with 2–3 eggs, ½–1 avocado, a handful of spinach, and a whole sliced tomato. Serve with ½–1 cup full-fat coconut milk.

- Pancakes: To ¾–1 cup (preferably) gluten-free flour or almond flour, add ½ teaspoon baking powder, 2–4 tablespoons whole full-fat coconut milk, 1 egg, 1 scoop rice, pea, or hemp protein powder (e.g., LivingProtein), 1 teaspoon vanilla, 1 teaspoon cinnamon, and 1–2 tablespoons raw honey. Add water to desired texture. Grill with coconut oil or butter.

- Bread with berry spread—Spread two slices gluten-free bread or a gluten-free wrap with one handful of fresh raspberries, strawberries, or blueberries. Add 1 handful of pumpkin seeds, walnuts, or almonds or spread with nut butter. Serve with 2 scoops protein powder stirred into 4–6 ounces full-fat coconut milk.

- Eating Out at a Restaurant—potatoes and fruit + eggs and bacon.

Snack 1:

- 1 piece fruit—recommend grapefruit, handful blueberries, pear, or green apple. For added calories, include a handful of nuts.
- 1 cup shake—see list at end of meal plan.
- 1 energy bar or snack mix—choose gluten-free bar or healthy snack mix. There is a list of snack mixes at the end of this chapter. Also one of my favorite resources for bars, snack mixes etc. is the website "Barefoot Provisions."
- Bell pepper and jicama strips with hummus (store-bought or homemade is fine—200-250 calories of hummus). How to make your own hummus: Blend 1 ½ cups of garbanzo beans (preferably rinsed and soaked), ½ cup tahini, 3 tablespoons olive oil, 1–2 shallots, ½ teaspoon sea salt, ½ teaspoon cumin, ½ teaspoon black pepper, ½ cup lemon

juice, 2 tablespoon chopped parsley, and a pinch of paprika. Serve a ½-cup sized portion with ½ sliced red and green pepper or 5–6 slices of jicama. Refrigerate the remainder. Add cayenne pepper for a metabolic boost. To improve digestibility, prior to cooking, soak the garbanzo beans for up to 24 hours and add just a bit of vinegar in the soaking solution.

Lunch:

(choose 1, can use kelp, kombu, or dulse seasoning)

- Wrap: For outer wrap, use gluten-free wrap. You could also use kale, bok choy, or some other large, dark leafy green, and then just include a brown or white rice inside wrap. For meat, use 4–6oz turkey, chicken, ground beef, ground buffalo, or non-fried fish. For vegetable options, use avocado, peppers, cucumber, tomato, sprouts, red onion, or celery. For sauce or dressing options, use olive oil/vinaigrette, lemon or lime juice, a soy sauce alternative, or a mix of all three.
- Turkey avocado sandwich or wrap. Use two slices gluten-free bread or wrap, 3–4 slices preservative-free, sodium-free deli turkey, ½–1 avocado, ½–1 tomato, 1 large handful dark leafy greens like spinach or kale.
- Cashew stir-fry: Cook 1 cup rice, quinoa, amaranth, or millet according to package directions. Sauté vegetables in 1 tablespoon sesame oil or coconut oil, adding: ½ sliced bell pepper, 1 teaspoon grated ginger root, 1 grated lime rind, 2 sliced shallots, 1 grated carrot, 1 handful sugar snap peas, 1 handful sliced mushrooms, 1 handful broccoli, 1 handful cashews, & ½ sliced cucumber. Spice with a pinch of turmeric & curry, then salt/pepper to taste. Serve 1–2 handfuls vegetable mix over ½–1 cup cooked starch.
- Sandwich—Good news: you can have a sandwich, but you just need to be careful to avoid modern grains and gut-irritating wheat. Preheat oven to 375.

While oven is heating, mix in a mixing bowl:

- 1/4 cup melted coconut oil
- 1/8 cup almond flour
- 1/4 cup protein powder
- 5 pastured eggs
- 1 tsp of sea salt
- 1 tsp of baking powder.

Spread this mixture thin on a greased baking sheet (brushing with olive oil is fine) and bake for 15 minutes and you will have bread done.

You can fill your sandwich with avocado; tomato; healthy meat of choice; an artisanal hard cheese such as parmesan, asiago, or gruyere; heathy mayo; salt; and pepper to taste.

To make mayo, simply blend

- 1 whole egg
- 1 Tbsp lemon juice
- salt and pepper
- while slowly adding 1 cup of olive oil, macadamia nut oil, or avocado oil (you'll see it thicken as you add oil).

- Leftovers: 1 serving from dinner

Snack 2:

- 1 handful snack mix—Choose 1 from list at end of this meal plan
- Guacamole: Blend ½ avocado and stir in ½ chopped red or green pepper, ½ chopped tomato, ½ teaspoon cumin, and a sprinkling of cayenne pepper. Serve with a 2–3 handfuls of gluten-free crackers or rice crackers, or for a lower calorie option, carrot sticks, jicama strips, or red or orange peppers.

Snack 3:

(during workout for longer workouts—or refer to "long workout fueling" section towards end of this book)

- Into water bottle during workouts: 3–4 tablespoons chia seeds or 1 tablespoon MCT oil, 1 tablespoon raw honey, 1 tablespoon electrolytes or sea salts, 5–10 grams amino acids. You can find plenty of suggestions/resources for electrolytes and amino acids here: (greenfieldfitnesssystems.com).
- 5–10g amino acids 30 minutes prior to and during your main workouts. Use BCAAs or EAAs (branched chain amino acids or essential amino acids—and the latter are far more complete and superior).
- During long workouts, a combination of Athlytes (you can also get those from Millennium Sports with 50% discount code MSTBG09) at 2 every 30 minutes + a fat-based energy gel of your choosing at 100–150 calories every 30 minutes + 5–10g amino acids every 60 minutes.
- Natural Force ISKIATE Endurance—1–2 servings per hour. You can get 10% discount with code BEN10 at NaturalForce website: (mynaturalforce.com/#bengreenfield).

Dinner:

- ***Beer Can Chicken and Black Quinoa & Kale salad***

Beer Can Chicken

- 1 (4 lbs) whole chicken
- 2 Tbsp coconut oil or grape seed oil
- 2 Tbsp salt
- 1 tsp black pepper
- 3 Tbsp of your favorite dry spice rub
- 1 can of beer

1. Remove neck and giblets from chicken and discard. Rinse chicken inside and out, and pat dry with paper towels. Rub chicken lightly with oil then rub inside and out with salt, pepper, and dry rub. Set aside.
2. Open a beer can and pour out half or drink half, whatever you prefer. Place beer can on a rimmed baking sheet. Place the chicken cavity over the beer can.
3. Cook the chicken at 350 degrees for approximately 1 ¼ hours or until the internal temperature registers 165 degrees F in the breast area and 180 degrees F in the thigh, or until the thigh juice runs clear when stabbed with a sharp knife. Remove from oven and let rest for 10 minutes before carving.

Black Quinoa & Kale Salad

- 1 ½ cups black quinoa cooked and cooled

Dressing:

- 4 Tbsp olive oil
- ½ organic lemon (peel and juice)
- 2 Tbsp hot mustard
- salt and pepper to taste

Salad:

- 4 big leaves of Kale
- 2 apples
- 1 handful of sprouts
- 1 cup of feta or goat cheese

Cook the quinoa. Mix the ingredients for the dressing in a tall glass or a small bowl. Let the quinoa cool off for a while and then add the dressing. Rinse and chop the kale. Cut the apples in small cubes. Mix all the ingredients with the quinoa and top it with the feta or goat cheese.

Barley Bean Soup

- 3 Tbsp olive oil
- 2 spring onions, chopped
- 3 cloves garlic, chopped
- 3 small carrots, diced
- 2 ribs celery, diced
- 2 tsp fresh rosemary, chopped
- 2 bay leaves (can be replaced with sage)
- juice from ½ lemon
- ½ glass white wine
- 8 cups vegetable stock or bone broth
- 1 cup pearled barley
- 1 zucchini, cut in quarters
- 10 cherry tomatoes, divided in half
- 2 cups fresh green beans
- 1 cup beans, soaked overnight and preboiled

Heat olive oil in a heavy-bottomed pot and add onion and garlic. Sauté for about 5 minutes. Add carrots, celery, rosemary, bay leaves, lemon juice, and white wine and cook, stirring often, for 2 minutes. Add vegetable stock and let it cook for 30 minutes. Add barley, zucchini, and tomatoes and let it cook for another 25 min. Then add green beans and beans and let it simmer for 10 more min. Remove the bay leaves and add salt and pepper. The soup is done when the barley and the beans are done. Serve with olive oil, lemon juice, and fresh herbs.

- ***Zucchini and Chickpeas Salad with Pancetta and Turkey Meatloaf***

Pancetta and Turkey Meatloaf (an adapted recipe from Giada De Laurentiis)

- ½ cup ground oats or gluten-free bread crumbs
- ½ cup chopped flat-leaf parsley
- 2 large eggs, lightly beaten
- 2 Tbsp whole milk
- ½ cup grated Romano or Parmesan cheese
- ¼ cup chopped sun-dried tomatoes
- ¾ tsp salt
- ¾ tsp freshly ground black pepper
- 1 pound ground turkey, preferably dark meat
- 10 ounces sliced pancetta, about 10 slices, or you can use bacon

1. Preheat the oven to 375 degrees F.
2. In a large bowl, stir together the oats or bread crumbs, parsley, eggs, milk, cheese, sun-dried tomatoes, salt, and pepper. Add the turkey and gently stir to combine, being careful not to overwork the meat.
3. On a baking sheet lined with parchment paper, lay out the pancetta, overlapping the slices, into a large rectangular shape. In the middle of the rectangle, place the turkey mixture, shaping it into a loaf. Using the parchment paper, wrap the pancetta up and around the turkey loaf to cover completely. Squeeze the parchment-covered loaf with your hands to secure the pancetta and solidify the shape of the loaf. While still covered in parchment, bake the loaf until the internal temperature reaches 165 degrees F on an instant-read thermometer, about 45 minutes. Remove from the oven and let cool.

- ***Zucchini and Chickpea Salad***

Dressing:

- 2 Tbsp fresh lemon juice
- ¼ cup olive oil
- ½ tsp salt
- ¼ tsp pepper

Combine all ingredients.

Salad:

- 1 cup cooked garbanzo beans, soaked
- 2 medium zucchini, cut into ¼-in pieces
- ½ cup frozen corn, thawed
- ½ small red onion, thinly sliced
- 1 red bell pepper, diced
- 1 oz parmesan cubed into ¼-in pieces

Place the garbanzo beans, zucchini, corn, red onion, and lettuce in a large salad bowl. Pour the vinaigrette over the salad and toss well. Garnish with the crumbled parmesan cheese and serve.

- ***Black Bean Flautas and Mexican Cabbage salad***

Black Bean Flautas

- 2 tsp coconut oil
- 1 medium onion, chopped (about 1 cup)
- 2 cloves garlic, minced (about 2 tsp)
- 2 cups black beans, rinsed and soaked
- 2 tsp chili powder
- 1 16-oz tub prepared salsa, divided
- 1 cup fresh or frozen corn kernels
- 12 6-inch sprouted gluten-free or corn tortillas
- ¼ cup chopped cilantro

1. Heat oil in skillet over medium heat. Cook onion 3 to 5 minutes, or until soft. Add garlic and cook 1 minute, or until translucent and fragrant.
2. Stir in beans, chili powder, and 1 cup water. Reduce heat to medium-low and simmer 10 minutes, or until most of the liquid has evaporated. Remove from heat. Mash beans until mixture is thickened but still chunky and some beans remain whole. Stir in 1 cup salsa and corn, and season with salt and pepper. Cool.
3. Preheat oven to 425F. Coat 2 large baking sheets with cooking spray. Spoon 1/3 cup black bean mixture down center of each tortilla. Roll tortilla around filling and secure closed with a toothpick. Set on prepared baking sheet. Repeat with remaining tortillas and black bean mixture. Bake 6 to 10 minutes, or until tortillas are browned and crisp.
4. Meanwhile, combine cilantro and remaining salsa in small bowl. Place 2 flautas on each plate and top with remaining salsa.

Mexican Cabbage Salad

- ½ head large cabbage, shredded
- ½ cup fresh cilantro, chopped
- ¼ cup fresh mint, chopped
- 1 medium cucumber, chopped

Honey Lime Dressing

- Juice of 1 lime
- ¼ cup olive oil
- 2 Tbsp raw honey
- 2 Tbsp finely chopped cilantro
- 1 garlic clove, peeled and minced (or 1 medium shallot, minced)
- ½ tsp kosher salt
- Freshly ground pepper

Combine ingredients and shake very well. Toss salad. Eat until full.

- ***Liver Pate:***

The recipe uses ½ lb of liver, so will be enough for 2–3 meals—and leftovers can be refrigerated for 2–3 days. Use organic liver only. Slice the liver into 1-cm (1/2-inch) thick pieces soak for 1–2 hours in milk (preferably organic, grass-fed milk). If you don't have milk or don't like milk, lemon juice is fine. Brown the liver slices in butter or ghee, cooking 3–4 minutes per side on low heat. At the same time, boil 1 egg. After liver is browned or while liver is browning, cook 1 diced onion for 5–10 minutes on same sauté pan.

Other ingredients are:

- an onion
- boiled egg
- 4 Tbsp butter
- plus a similar amount of coconut oil;
- cilantro (or you can use kimchi in place of the cilantro, for a spicier flavor).

1. Put everything—the cooked liver, cooked onion, cooking fluids from the pot, and boiled egg, along with 2 tablespoons coconut oil, and a handful of fresh chopped cilantro—into a blender and purée.
2. Serve the pate with rice crackers, flax seed crackers, or wrapped in bok choy, Swiss chard, nori or butter lettuce. If you don't use crackers, serve with 1 baked sweet potato or yam, over a bed of mixed greens.

- **Restaurant**: Splurge at your favorite restaurant. Order a clean, organic, grass-fed or wild-caught protein (e.g. steak or fish) with a clean carbohydrate (e.g., white rice, mashed sweet potato, regular sweet potato or regular potato, quinoa) and a side vegetable that is as dark and colorful as possible (e.g. kale, spinach, etc.). As a side order, any sulfur-rich vegetable on the menu (Brussel sprouts, onions, garlic, broccoli, cauliflower, etc.) Travel with sea salt if you can and salt liberally. Leave any sauces off and get olive oil or coconut oil on side if they have it. Try to avoid things that were cooked in vegetables oils and things that contain a high amount of non-nutrient dense starches (e.g., going to a Mexican restaurant and mowing through two baskets of fried chips).

Desserts and Cheat Meals:

(consume before, during, or after exercise only, preferably only three days of the week)

- EnergyBits—Eat 50-100 EnergyBits (pop them like popcorn). Use 10% discount code "BEN": (energybits.com)
- ***Coconut-Chocolate-Chia Blend***

In a small bowl, mix:

- 25–50 EnergyBits
- 2 tsp carob or cocoa powder
- 4–6oz full-fat coconut milk
- 2–3 tablespoons chia seeds or unsweetened coconut flakes.

Stir and chill in refrigerator for 15–20 minutes. For added crunch, throw on some unsweetened coconut flakes.

- ***Sea Salt, Dark Chocolate and Almonds***

Use about a quarter bar of a good dark chocolate, then toss it into a small bowl with a handful of raw almonds 2–3 pinches of sea salt, preferably the mind-glowingly good Aztecan sea salt. I pop this like popcorn, often during a good flick. For added kick, include a pinch of cayenne pepper.

- ***Protein Parfait***

Into 1 scoops of organic whey or vegan protein
add full-fat coconut milk to desired texture, along with

  - 1 tsp almond butter
  - a handful of unsweetened coconut flakes
  - 1 tsp of cinnamon.

I typically stir, rather than blending, and eat with a spoon at approximately ice cream/custard texture.

- ***Healthy Chocolate Pudding***

Blend together:

  - ½ sliced avocado
  - 1 tsp cinnamon
  - 1 scoop of organic whey or vegan protein
  - 4–6oz full-fat coconut milk
  - 1 tsp almond butter
  - 1–2 tsp carob or cocoa powder
  - a dash of natural vanilla extract or vanilla powder.

- ***Dipped Dark Chocolate***

On ½ a bar, drizzle a tablespoon of raw almond or cashew butter, or simply dip the chocolate bar in the jar of raw nut butter.

Snack Mix Recipes:

- **Berry Almond Snack Mix:** Mix at beginning of week: 2 cups almonds, 1 cup dried cherries or blueberries, 1 cup flax seeds. Keep in freezer.
- **Sunny Seed Mix (highest in iron):** Mix at beginning of week: 3 cups sunflower seeds, 1 cup sesame seeds, 1 cup pumpkin seeds, 1 cup flax seeds. Keep in freezer.
- **Tropical Snack Mix (also very high in iron):** Mix at beginning of week: 2 cups raw coconut shavings (preferably unsweetened), 2 cups raisins or Craisins, 2 cups Brazil nuts, 1 cup dried mango or chopped papaya, and 1 cup flax seeds. Keep in freezer.

Shake Recipes:

For higher calories or post-workout shakes, I highly recommend adding 10–20 grams of LivingProtein or DEEP30 Whey Protein. Any shakes with fruit are only to be consumed on carb refeed day or as a quick substitute for dinners on the other days of the week.

- **Blueberry Coconut Shake:** Combine a handful of frozen blueberries; 3 tablespoons of shredded, unsweetened coconut; and ice to desired texture. Add approximately 4oz unsweetened full-fat coconut milk or full-fat, organic yogurt (if completely necessary, for this and the following shakes, you can use unsweetened almond milk, rice milk, or water, but this is not as good as coconut milk or yogurt) to desired texture and blend.
- **Nutty Shake:** Combine 1 tablespoon almond butter; 2 tablespoons shredded, unsweetened coconut; 2 tablespoons sunflower seeds; ice; and 4oz water or, unsweetened full-fat coconut milk, or yogurt, almond milk, or rice milk.

- **Coconut-Kiwi:** Blend together 4oz unsweetened full-fat coconut milk, almond milk, rice milk, or water, ½ cup frozen apricots or peaches; and 1 frozen kiwi.
- **Berry Shake:** Combine a handful of frozen berries and ice to desired texture. Add 4oz unsweetened full-fat coconut milk, yogurt, almond milk, rice milk, or water, and blend.
- **Nutty Banana Shake:** Combine 2 tablespoons flax seeds, 1 handful almonds or walnuts, 1 banana, and ice to desired texture. Add 4oz unsweetened full-fat coconut milk, yogurt, almond milk, rice milk, or water.

Long Workout "Real Food" Options

Important: When I say "long workout," I'm referring to workouts that are A) relatively tough and not just an "aerobic walk" or easy hike; and B) 2+ hours. An example would be a multi-hour hard Ironman-prep bike ride; a hard, weighted day hike; an interval-based trail run, etc. Unless you're completely fasted going into the workout and it's a tough workout close to an hour, you do not really need to fuel during your workouts for anything other than the situation described in A or B.

For example, these are the type of workouts you'd do during training for a big endurance race, during some type of triathlon or cycling camp, or for a tough weekend workout.

The goal is to consume 150-300 calories per hour if you are female or a small individual or 250-400 calories per hour if you are male or a large individual, and to get these from sources that are not pure sugar.

Choices are:

- **2-3 handfuls of snack mix per hour (see recipes earlier in this plan)**
- **Chia seed/water/electrolyte mix—24–32 ounces per hour.**

Instructions:

1. Put ⅓ cup of dry chia seeds into a 32-ounce Nalgene or other water bottle.
2. Fill the Nalgene with water a third of the way and then pour chia seeds into the water.
3. Add 1–2 teaspoons of a good sea salt (I like Aztecan)
4. Close the lid tightly and shake the bottle, then open the bottle and fill it with water the rest of the way. Close the lid and shake again.
5. To prevent lumps from forming, shake about every 5 minutes.
6. Add stevia and lemon if desired for sweetness.

- **Carob Cashew Bars—2-3/hr**
  - 1 cup cashew butter
  - 2–3 Tbsp honey
  - 1 ½ cups protein powder (check GreenfieldFitnessSystems.com for my favorite whey and vegan options)
  - 1 cup old fashioned, gluten-free oats
  - 1 Tbsp carob powder

Mix the cashew butter and honey in a bowl and heat for 30 seconds (use a saucepan, or in a pinch, a microwave). Add the rest of the ingredients and mix together. Mixture should be crumbly. Press (hard) into a 9x9 tray and refrigerate for 20 minutes. Cut into bars.

- **Chocolate Almond Butter "Rollies"—equivalent of 1–2 wraps per hour**

Spread 1 tablespoon of almond butter, 1 teaspoon honey, and 2 tablespoons carob chips or chocolate chips into a sprouted wrap, roll up, and chop into bite-size pieces. Carry in aluminum foil.

- **The Get-Fit Guy Superfood Bar**

Here is the recipe (inspired by this article on the best ingredients for energy bars): (http://bit.ly/1Hwl6P3)

Ingredients:

- 1 cup cashews
- 1 cup goji berries
- ½ cup chia seeds (preferably soaked)
- ½ cup spirulina or chlorella powder
- ½ cup cacao powder
- ⅓ cup rolled oats
- 2 Tbsp raw honey or, for lower sugar version, 1 tsp stevia
- 1 Tbsp coconut oil, melted

- 2 Tbsp hemp seeds
- 4 Tbsp maca root powder
- 1 Tbsp dulse, kelp, or sea salt

Instructions:

1. Line an 8-inch baking pan with parchment paper and set aside.
2. Pulse cashews in food processor until crumbly, place in a separate bowl.
3. Pulse goji berries in food processor until finely chopped. Add all other ingredients to the goji berry mixture and process until well combined. If goji berries are a bit too spendy for you, you can use dried apricots instead.
4. Add the chopped cashews to the mixture and pulse until well combined.
5. Firmly press the entire mixture into the baking pan, using the flat surface of a measuring cup to create a flat even layer.
6. Place pan in the freezer for one hour, then remove and cut into 8 rectangular bars (or more or less, depending on desired size).
7. Place in an airtight container and store for up to one month in the fridge.

Power Protein Bars

Ingredients:

- 2 cups raw or slightly roasted almonds
- ½ cup ground flax seeds, chia seeds, or pumpkin seeds
- ½ cup raisins, currants, dried dates
- ½ cup shredded unsweetened coconut
- ½ cup unsalted peanut or almond butter
- ½ cup melted coconut oil
- 2 tsp vanilla extract
- ½ tsp sea salt

- 3 T honey
- 4 ounces dark chocolate—optional

Instructions:

Prepare the almonds, flax seeds, dried fruit, and coconut by processing them in the food processor until they are coarsely ground. Add almond butter and salt and mix. In a small saucepan, melt coconut oil over low heat until it becomes liquid. Stir in honey and vanilla extract. Combine the melted coconut oil with the nuts and fruit, working with a few pulses in the food processor until it forms a coarse paste. Spoon the mixture into the 8 x 8-inch baking dish, letting it chill for 1 hour in the refrigerator. Using a small saucepan melt the chocolate over low heat, stirring frequently so that the chocolate does not burn. When melted, spread over the bars and return the baking dish to the refrigerator for an additional 30 minutes, or until the chocolate hardens. Cut into bars, then wrap individual bars in freezer paper, or wax paper. Store in cool, dry area or freeze.

When it comes to eating real food during a workout, there are a multitude of other options, and the book "Real Food Recipes For Your Long Workouts" reveals even more options, but the list above includes some of my favorites and will hopefully get your wheels turning!

Race Week

Up to the point where you reach the week of your big event, you have been on a fairly low carbohydrate intake, but you don't want to go into your event in a state of complete storage carbohydrate (glycogen) depletion.

So you have a few options. For a very long race (Ironman or longer) or a multi-day event (a long adventure race), you can begin about five to six days prior to your event to gradually fuel with more carbohydrate. For a shorter race, such as a 90+ minute event, you only need to slightly increase carbohydrate intake two to three days prior to the event. For anything less than 90 minutes, there's really no need to change up your regular nutrition routine at all, aside from eating a prerace meal containing slightly higher-than-normal carbohydrate levels if you're not planning on implementing full ketosis for the event.

Let's use a longer race and a longer carb load as an example. We'll use a Sunday race for this example.

Beginning Monday or Tuesday on the week of your race, add the equivalent of one large sweet potato or yam with an egg-based breakfast, or switch to one of the "power" cereal breakfast recipes found in the meal plan earlier in this book, or begin adding fruit to your morning smoothie.

Also beginning Monday or Tuesday on the week of your race, include a side of ¾ –1 cup cooked wild rice, white rice, or mashed sweet potato or yam with your lunchtime salad. Salt and pepper to taste, and if you'd like, you can even boil or roast vegetables and serve those over the rice instead of having your extra carbohydrates with a cold salad. The idea is to naturally include just a little extra carbohydrate with both breakfast and lunch, rather than following the typical scenario of saving all of your carbohydrates for your evening meal.

Your evening meal isn't going to change much since you already have been including the majority of the day's carbohydrates with your evening meal. So the only thing you're really changing is adding a little bit of extra carbohydrate to breakfast and to lunch. If you're concerned about the health effects of an entire week of a post-meal spike in blood glucose after multiple meals, then you can use a pre-meal supplement such as bitter melon extract to decrease the rise in blood glucose.

You'll also want to pay more attention to not going hungry after your workouts during the week of the race, and this will mean timing your workouts to end no more than 20 minutes prior to your breakfast, lunch, or dinner, or placing more priority on a post-workout snack such as a piece of raw fruit, chunks of cooked sweet potato or yam, a few handfuls of berries of your choice blended with ice, a serving of rice, etc.

For dinner the night before your big event, I recommend:

- 2 digestive enzymes prior to the meal.
- 1 large or 2 medium sweet potatoes or yams served with mineral dense sea salt (e.g. Aztec salt) along with coconut oil or olive oil. Another clean-burning starch alternative is white rice. For any of these options, boil or bake—don't fry.
- 1 bed of iron rich leafy greens, boiled or steamed. Dinosaur kale is a good choice, as is spinach, bok choy, or any dark leafy green. For this, you can also add coconut oil or olive oil and sea salt.
- Wild-caught salmon or grass-fed beef, 6–8 ounces, prepared as desired.
- 1 glass of red wine.
- ½ a bar of "healthy dark" chocolate.

The next morning, your prerace meal, as you have probably guessed, should be a complex carbohydrate that is easily digested, and my top recommendation is either:

- 1–2 medium-large sweet potatoes or yams with salt, 1 tablespoon honey or maple syrup, and a dab of almond butter or . . .
- 400–600 calories of white rice with olive oil and sea salt. Try to have this meal completely finished at least two hours and no more than three hours before the race begins. If you really want to delve into the nitty-gritty science and math behind this approach, take a listen to or read Part 1: (quickanddirtytips.com/getfitguy244) and Part 2: (quickanddirtytips.com/getfitguy245) of my Get-Fit Guy series on prerace meals.

I must emphasize that it's important to understand that the recommendations I have just given are for carbohydrate loading prior to a big, voluminous, somewhat intense, daylong or multi-day event. This is the only scenario the entire training and racing year during which you need to eat this amount of carbohydrates, and I will readily admit that even in this scenario, this amount of carbohydrates is still more than what I would consider to be "healthy." However, if you've been "training low carb" the rest of the year, you can vastly increase your glycogen stores with the method I've just described.

In simple terms, all you're really doing is naturally replacing some of your primarily fat- and protein-based meals with carbohydrates.

For a shorter event (an event that is 90+ minutes, but less than a full day), you can use the exact approach I've just outlined, but the increase in carbohydrate intake only needs to occur for 2–3 days and not for 5–6 days prior to the event.

Finally, allow me to once again remind you that the scenario I've just outlined is not a scenario you'd use if you were trying to follow "strict ketosis" and stay in a completely ketogenic state for your race. Ultimately, strict ketosis can be difficult for many folks to follow and can result in an energy bonk during your event if you're not extremely fat adapted and using very large amounts of amino acids and medium chain triglycerides during your event. For most athletes, I'm a bigger fan of going low carb or "cycling ketogenic" during the entire training year, then shifting to slightly higher carb intake for a brief period of time during race week. The added advantage of this approach is that if you've kept yourself in a low-carb state much of the year, your body will readily soak up these extra race week carbohydrates as storage glycogen, and you'll store away more carbs than you would under normal circumstances.

Race Day

Before jumping into what to eat during your big event, and some sample eating scenarios, let's first begin by looking at some things that you simply shouldn't eat before you're about to ask your body to perform at the highest level. Some of these will directly decrease performance by creating bloating and gas or by drawing precious blood away from your muscles and into your gut. And some will allow you to perform just fine but will make you feel like crap after you're done—or that night, or the next day, or a decade later after your gut is destroyed by years of accumulative unhealthy fueling.

There are five common dietary errors I see athletes make prior to hitting it hard, so here's what to avoid:

1) FODMAPs like fructose and maltodextrin.

FODMAPs can be a leading cause of gut rot, GI distress, gas, bloating, diarrhea and constipation if you eat a bunch of them before you exercise or race. Go here to read up on FODMAPs, then—especially if you've been experiencing stomach issues—avoid them: (http://bit.ly/1Ork9J7). Three big FODMAPs I see lots of athletes including in prerace meals are wheat, dairy, and fermentable fruits like apples and pears. Many popular sports nutrition compounds also include high amounts of fructose and/or maltodextrin. These are not a good idea, especially if you have a sensitive stomach.

2) High amounts of caffeine.

Caffeine can enhance sports performance. But that doesn't mean more is better—especially if you're concerned about your long-term adrenal health or the chances of overworking your central nervous system.

Most recommendations you'll find in sports nutrition literature tell you to eat about 0.5–1.5 mg caffeine per pound of body weight (that's about 1–3 mg per kg). For a 150-lb (68-kg) athlete, that's a dose of 70–210 mg of caffeine. But I recommend you choose the minimum amount possible because when caffeine intake gets too high or goes on for too long, there is an increase in side effects like jitteriness, nervousness, insomnia, headache, dizziness, and gastrointestinal distress, all of which can impair your athletic performance or cause long-term adrenal issues.

3) Artificial sweeteners and chemical cocktails

One common artificial sweetener found in sports nutrition supplements is sugar alcohol—which is a FODMAP. Another common one is sucralose, which can damage the good bacteria in your GI tract. Many others, such as aspartame and acesulfame potassium are neurotoxic and can cause brain fog while you're exercising. So I highly recommend you avoid all of the above prior to exercise. You'll be surprised once you begin inspecting labels at how many sports nutrition fuels actually include the stuff. Of course, there are chemicals that go above and beyond just artificial sweeteners. Take Ensure for example. It is a common prerace meal for Ironman triathletes and marathoners, and the ingredients consist of:

Milk Protein Concentrate, Canola Oil, Soy Protein Concentrate, Corn Oil, Short-Chain Fructooligosaccharides, Whey Protein Concentrate, Magnesium Phosphate, Natural and Artificial Flavors, Potassium Citrate, Sodium Citrate, Soy Lecithin, Calcium Phosphate, Potassium Chloride, Salt (Sodium Chloride), Choline Chloride, Ascorbic Acid, Carrageenan, Ferrous Sulfate, dl-Alpha-Tocopheryl Acetate, Zinc Sulfate, Niacinamide, Manganese Sulfate, Calcium Pantothenate,

Cupric Sulfate, Vitamin A Palmitate, Thiamine Chloride Hydrochloride, Pyridoxine Hydrochloride, Riboflavin, Folic Acid, Chromium Chloride, Biotin, Sodium Molybdate, Sodium Selenate, Potassium Iodide, Phylloquinone, Vitamin D3, and Cyanocobalamin.

If there are over a dozen ingredients you can barely even pronounce, it's usually a pretty good sign your body is going to have difficulty digesting it during a workout, or that it might not be that great for your long-term health. You can read more about my beef with Ensure and other so-called "health foods" for athletes in this blog article, in which I talk about why these things are also a fast track to the average person getting fat: (http://bit.ly/1EYQtkw).

4) High amounts of fiber.

Fiber is not only primarily digested in your colon, but it also significantly slows gastric emptying, so consuming too much fiber before a workout simply results in a lot of undigested foodstuff in your stomach and intestine. Big bowls of pre-workout or prerace fiber enriched cereals, oatmeal, fruit smoothies and kale shakes can cause some serious issues, especially for long workouts—so be careful. Incidentally, I've found from personal experience that I can go pound the pavement hard within as little as an hour after downing a well-blended kale smoothie, while the same amount of kale in a salad leaves me feeling less than stellar. So blending (or juicing) can help you get some of the phytonutrients without requesting as much work from your digestive system.

5) Heavy, non-portable foods.

If your goal is speed or aerodynamics, then giant sweet potatoes, bananas, water-filled fruits, and melted dark chocolate bars are not a great solution. There are right ways to consume real food during your workout (which you're about to learn). But there are also wrong ways to consume real food during your workout—and if something is big, bulky, and heavy it's going to inhibit your performance.

So what kind of strategies *do* I recommend for eating before your workout or race? Assuming that we're talking about a glycogen-depleting effort of 1.5+ hours in duration (which is really the only time you'll get a significant performance enhancing benefit out of eating a meal before your race) here are the top five things to include before a workout or race:

1) Blended & juiced foods.

When you blend or juice foods, you make things much easier on your digestive system, allowing foods to empty more quickly from the stomach. Blending or juicing also helps to predigest the food so your body doesn't have to work as hard during digestion. This frees up precious energy for you to be able to devote to breathing, moving, and contracting muscles. Cell walls are broken down and nutrients are quickly released (especially from greens like kale, or dark root vegetables like beets and carrots.) When you use these strategies, you're essentially "chewing" your food much more thoroughly than you may have been able to with your teeth, and many foods that would normally have given you digestive trouble—such as a bunch of carrots or a big spinach salad—will digest just fine when blended or juiced. I recommend a high-speed, quality blender such as a Vitamix, an Omega masticating juicer, and a Magic Bullet for travel. Two of my "go-to" recipes for pre-workout are a kale smoothie blended with coconut water or coconut milk, or a carrot-ginger-lemon juice with a touch of olive oil added in.

2) Small amounts of caffeine.

As you learned earlier, caffeine can definitely help with sports performance. 1,3,7-trimethylxanthine, more popularly known as caffeine, is the world's most consumed natural pharmacological agent. Caffeine has been shown to improve endurance and time-trial performance in cyclists, increase endurance in runners, and improve performance times and boost power in rowers. Caffeine has also been shown to improve performance in cycling and running events lasting five minutes or more, and to increase power output, speed, and strength in sprint and power events lasting less than ten seconds (incidentally, caffeine has been shown to have no effect, and may even be a negative factor, in sprint and power events lasting anywhere from fifteen seconds to three minutes)

In tennis players, caffeine increases hitting accuracy, speed and agility, and overall success on the court. And players reported feeling more energy late in their matches. Caffeine also reduces your "rating of perceived exertion," or how hard you feel like you're actually working—which essentially causes you to push harder and faster.

Unfortunately, most people are averaging 238 mg of caffeine every day—which is the equivalent of 2–3 cups of coffee—and 20–30% of people consume an enormous 600 mg of caffeine daily (with about 71% of it coffee, 16% from tea, and 12% from soft drinks and energy drinks). And when we shove high amounts of caffeine into our system prior to a workout or race, it's just extra stress on the adrenal glands. So as mentioned earlier, I recommend a minimum effective dose of caffeine—about 0.5mg per pound of body weight or 1mg per kg of body weight. For a 150lb athlete that's the equivalent of a small cup of coffee.

3) Easy-to-digest carbohydrates.

White potato, sweet potato, yam, taro, and white rice are the top five carbohydrate sources that seem to be best tolerated by athletes prior to hard workouts. But if you're adhering to the carbohydrate/fat/protein ratios recommended earlier, then you know you don't even need ample amounts of these. How much do you actually need?

Let's say you wake up on race morning, and you've primarily burnt through your liver's glycogen stores while sleeping. The average human needs (at most) about 400 calories of carbohydrate to completely top off those stores (assuming you haven't been starving yourself, your muscles are already full of glycogen and ready to rumble). So if you eat 100 grams from any of the starch sources mentioned above, that's all you need. To put that number into context, that's about 2 cups of cooked white rice, or a couple large, boiled sweet potatoes or yams. Liberally add sea salt to either of the foods above, throw in a few tablespoons of the healthy fats and proteins you'll learn about momentarily, and you have a perfect pre-Ironman or pre-marathon meal!

And as you may already know, 400 calories of carbohydrate is much less than the recommended values of anywhere from 600-1500 calories!

If you're adhering to a strict ketogenic diet, you'll need even fewer carbohydrates than that, and for your pre-workout or prerace meal, you can simply get away with the minimum amount of carbohydrate necessary to keep your brain's neurons firing so that you don't lose mental function. This comes out to about 30 grams, or 120 calories of carbohydrate. Because ketosis produces this state of fat-utilizing metabolic efficiency, most of the athletes I've worked with who are implementing ketosis go into their big workout or race with a pre-event meal of Bulletproof Coffee, or a Ketogenic Kale Shake, or 1-2 servings of UCAN SuperStarch in coconut milk (more on SuperStarch later).

4) Easy-to-digest fats.

In contrast to fats that take a long time to digest, such as eggs, bacon, cheese or yogurt, medium chain triglycerides from sources such as MCT oil, coconut oil or the solid form of coconut manna actually bypass the normal process of digestion and instead get absorbed directly into your liver—where they can then be metabolized to provide a quick source of energy. This makes MCT's a valuable addition to your "before" meal. For joint and heart health, you can also include small amounts of a concentrated source of anti-inflammatory omega-3 essential fatty acids from a cold-press plant-based oil such as Udo's Oil or Panaseeda Five Oil Blend (you can simply include these in your smoothie or pour them over the top of your carbohydrate source). In particular, the Panaseeda blend actually was able to address a serious gut malabsorption issue in former Olympian & gold medal winner Andreas Wecker, completely healing his abdominal issues, and transforming him from a lifeless 78-pound man given only two hours to live. You can read about that story here: (http://bit.ly/1M7F55z).

5) Easy-to-digest proteins.

Like many fats, proteins also take a long time to digest and require lots of energy to break down—which is why a prerace meal of steak and eggs is a recipe for gut disaster or subpar performance. But for efforts of greater than three hours in duration, your body can use up to 15% of its energy requirements from protein. In addition, high blood levels of amino acid during exercise can lower your rating of perceived exertion and significantly decrease post-exercise soreness.

For this reason, I recommend that prior to your big workout or race you include any or all of the following: A) 20–30 grams of a hydrolyzed whey protein, which is a type of "pre-digested" protein that is more expensive but much easier to absorb and assimilate compared to regular whey protein (I recommend Mt. Capra's DEEP30 protein); B) 5–10 grams of an essential amino acids capsule or powder, which has an extremely high protein absorption rate C) 10–20 grams of a hydrolyzed collagen protein source. For this, I recommend you either use an organic, clean powder such as Great Lakes or Bernard Jensen, or simply drink a cup of bone broth with your prerace meal.

Compared to eating a steak, these type of protein sources will be far less stressful for your digestive system to break down and absorb. Remember—you don't want to be making your gut work any harder than it needs to.

Next, let's move into what may be the most common question I ever get: what should I eat during my race? This is an especially important question if you aren't going to go the traditional route of concentrated sports drinks, gels, sugary bars, chomps, chews, bloks, and jelly beans.

The good news is that there are healthy race-day fueling strategies that work quite well and also achieve an ideal balance of performance and health. Neither of these scenarios are 100% "ancestral" or what I consider to be completely ideal from a healthy human macronutrient intake standpoint, but let's face it—hammering on a bicycle for 100 miles is not exactly ancestral either. So the trick is to gently nudge your body towards primarily tapping into its own fatty acids as a fuel, or to present your body with as natural a fuel source as possible (e.g., white rice, bacon, eggs, etc.). You're about to learn both techniques.

This first scenario is ideal if you want to maximize your use of your body's natural and preferred fuel stores (fatty acids) while minimizing the rate at which you deplete your storage carbohydrates (glycogen). It simply involves eating moderate amounts of slow-release carbohydrates with small additions of easy-to-digest fats and amino acids.

It allows for extreme metabolic efficiency and fat burning with minimal gastric distress, and is my preferred mode of fueling for myself and any athletes I work with who desire to gain the health and fat-burning effects from lower carbohydrate intake or ketosis.

Here is what you need to pull it off:

6) Slow-release carbohydrate.

Ideally, an optimal carbohydrate source for athletes should have a low osmolality (to avoid those pregnant-mother carbohydrates from releasing all their babies mid-flight), with a slow time-release to avoid rapid fluctuations in glucose and blood-sugar spikes or crashes. To my knowledge, there is currently only one carbohydrate source that exists that satisfies this scenario: a product called "SuperStarch," which is made by UCAN.

Contrary to popular belief among athletes and coaches who I've spoken to about this unique starch, SuperStarch is not a sugar or a fiber. Chemically it is a complex carbohydrate or starch that is completely absorbed. It is an extremely large glucose chain with a molecular weight between 500,000 and 700,000 g/mol.

What does it mean to have a high molecular weight? Since molecular weight and osmolality are inversely related, SuperStarch exerts a very low osmotic pressure in the gastrointestinal tract. This means it is rapidly emptied from your stomach into your intestines, which means it is very gentle on your gut.

When it reaches your intestines, SuperStarch is semi-resistant to digestion, but is eventually completely absorbed into the bloodstream, which gives it a slow time-release absorption profile. Because of this slow rate of release, your body taps into its own fatty acids as a fuel source, and you need about half as many carbohydrates as you would normally consume (e.g., if you were accustomed to consuming three gels per hour, you would only consume about one serving, or 100 calories, of SuperStarch per hour).

The only issue with SuperStarch is that it can create digestive distress in some folks. If you try it, and you get gas, bloating, etc., then in my opinion the next best option for a relatively slow release or lower sugar sports nutrition fueling powder is ISKIATE Endurance fuel, made by Natural Force (use code BEN10 to save 10%).

7) Easy-to-digest fats.

Since the seed-based oils I mentioned earlier are not very heat stable, your top choices for fats will be either MCT oil or coconut oil. You can definitely go overboard with either. Research shows that consuming more than about ten grams per hour over the course of a multi-hour exercise session can lead gastric distress. In the case of MCT oil, ten grams is about the equivalent of one tablespoon. So you would add one tablespoon per hour to the one serving of SuperStarch or ISKIATE per hour. Some larger male athletes can handle slightly more MCT oil and SuperStarch than this, but you need to experiment by starting with one tablespoon and one serving.

8) Easy-to-digest amino acids.

To your bottle, which already contains the SuperStarch or ISKIATE and easy-to-digest fats, you add either ten grams of a hydrolyzed whey protein for each hour of exercise, or five to ten grams of essential amino acids capsule or powder, or ten grams of a hydrolyzed collagen protein source. You mix this with the fats and the SuperStarch or ISKIATE into one bottle. If you really want to live life on the edge, you can throw in an all-natural amino acid complex derived from the Asian Mandarin Vespa Wasp, which works by shifting the muscles to metabolize a higher level of fat.

And that's it. You can mix all this in a slightly less dense solution in a water bottle that can be used for multi-hour fueling, or in a dense concentrated solution in a flask for activities such as running and hiking.

Finally, SuperStarch, ISKIATE, and many other powders tend to "clump" and settle in the bottom of your bottle. To avoid this, it can be helpful to:

1. Mix this brew at the last possible hour, and stir and shake vigorously.
2. Consider blending everything in a blender and putting into a wide mouth "Floe" bottle (which also allows you to add ice if you're racing in hot conditions).
3. Put in small amounts of an electrolyte powder or electrolyte capsules into the bottle, which tends to reduce clumping.

Now, here's a caveat to everything you've just read: there are some situations in which using a liquid fueling scenario like the one I just described simply doesn't work, or situations in which your liquid fueling needs to be accompanied by other fuel sources. These situations include:

1. Liquids need to be carried in either flasks or water bottles, and I've found that when doing races such as a Spartan or obstacle course event (in which you're often rolling or crawling on the ground) flasks and water bottles get smashed, leak, and can press up against your body in very uncomfortable ways.
2. Sometimes you need a "break" from the texture of liquids, and especially during long events such as an

Ironman triathlon, you may find you need either something to chew on, or something that has more of a gel-like texture.

3. Pre-made gels require no previous forethought, planning or mixing. You just put them in your pocket and . . . go.

Fortunately, when it comes to venturing outside of the realm of glucose, fructose, maltodextrin, honey and the other common sources of sugar used to form the base of most gels, there are a variety of fat-based energy gel options. You can go here to read an article I wrote in which you will find 12 fat-based alternatives to sickeningly sweet sugar-based sport gels: (http://bit.ly/1NzOwxN)

If you don't care for the texture of gels, and you don't have the time to make real food, you can also use "safe," gluten-free, soy- and lactose-free energy bars such as the Cocochia Bar, Hammer Recovery Bar, Hammer Vegan Recovery Bar, LaraBar, Nogii Bar, Quest Bar, Zing Bar, BonkBreaker Bar, or HeathWarrior Bar. At the time this book is being written, I'm even developing my own high-fat, low-carb energy bar over at GreenfieldFitnessSystems.com, so be sure to check there too!

Remember that the goal is not to use bottles full of dense energy or packets of gels or calorie-dense energy bars in all your training sessions. In most situations, you'll only use the type of race-day fueling scenario you've been reading about during a race, or once every couple weeks to "train your gut" during a training session. Otherwise, you can either exercise fasted with water only, or simply eat real food, such as trail mixes, chia seed slurries, pemmican, jerky, spirulina, or chlorella tablets, etc.

Liquids vs. Solids

But wait . . . isn't there an issue with using real food–based solids during exercise? After all, we've all been taught that when the going gets tough in a workout or race, liquids beat solids hands down, right?

To see if this is true, let's break down a March 2010 study in the Journal of Medicine and Science in Sports & Exercise, entitled "Oxidation of Solid versus Liquid Carbohydrate Sources":

Here's how the intro reads:

"The ingestion of carbohydrate (CHO) solutions has been shown to increase CHO oxidation and improve endurance performance. However, the majority of studies have investigated CHO in solution and sporting practice includes ingestion of CHO in solid (e.g., energy bars) as well as liquid form. It remains unknown whether CHO in solid form is as effectively oxidized as compared to CHO solutions."

So the researchers then went on to study cyclists who worked out for a three-hour aerobic cycling session. Here is what they found:

"The present study demonstrates that a GLU+FRC (glucose + fructose) mix administered as a solid BAR during cycling can lead to high mean and peak exogenous CHO (carbohydrate) oxidation rates (>1g/min). The GLU+FRC mix ingested in form of a solid BAR resulted in similar average and peak exogenous CHO oxidation rates and showed similar oxidation efficiencies as a DRINK. These findings suggest that CHO from a solid BAR is effectively oxidized during exercise and can be a practical form of supplementation alongside other forms of CHO."

Short and sweet summary: the solid bars did just as well as the liquids. *At least for cyclists.*

Additional studies—along with lots of anecdotal evidence among professional cyclists–has backed up this idea. So while it's established that when you're doing non-jarring, non-impact, non-weight bearing exercise like cycling, you can chomp away on real food if you don't feel like drinking liquids, what about for more stomach-sloshing motions like running?

Here's an interesting study on triathletes: (www.ncbi.nlm.nih.gov/pubmed/7751072) that gives us a good answer. In the study, Scientists at University of Utrecht in the Netherlands compared liquid versus solid carbohydrate intake before and during prolonged exercise in 32 triathletes who were training for at least a sprint triathlon. Study participants took part in hard workouts that consisted of two bouts of cycling lasting 45-50 minutes at about 75% VO2max (85% of maximum heart rate) and two running workouts lasting 45 minutes, also at 75% VO2max (Peters).

So first, the triathlete cycled, and then they ran. Then after a six-minute rest, they completed a maximal cycling test consisting of three minutes of pedaling at 175 Watts and then three minutes of 100% all-out intensity.

After four minutes of rest, the triathlete then cycled *again,* rested for six minutes, did a second maximal test on the bike, rested for four more minutes, then ran again, rested for six minutes, and then completed a final cycling test. If you were doing the math, that is over three hours of exercise with an average heart rate at or above 85% of maximum heart rate.

As if that weren't enough, each participant had to do this three times through at different times, each time with a different fueling scenario: once with caloric liquids only, once with a mix of solids and liquids (white bread, marmalade, and bananas—yum), and once with a non-caloric liquid placebo that was basically just food coloring. Water intake was the same between all groups.

So which treatment was best? Half of the triathletes in the study were able to complete all three hours of hard exercise when they took in liquids only, but only nine of the triathletes could handle the same workout once solids were added in. And even the ones who didn't finish the workout weren't able to go as hard for the part of the workout that they actually did complete.

In other words, once you introduce the stomach sloshing of hard running (think 10K to marathon, not slow jogs or ultra-runs) liquids beat solids hands down.

Take-away message: solids are just as good as liquids when you're riding a bike or doing non-impact activity, but once you start jarring the body and sloshing the stomach, try to stick to liquids (and I would actually consider a gel just as good as liquid, although there are no studies yet that look at that in runners).

Water & Electrolytes

Of course, no discussion of race day fueling would be complete without considering hydration and electrolyte needs. It was in the podcast interview "How You're Being Manipulated By The Sports Drink Industry And What You Can Do About It" with Dr. Tim Noakes that my paradigms were first shattered when it came to a new view of electrolyte intake.

In the interview, Dr. Noakes introduces an argument against the worldwide brainwashing that has been done by the Gatorade Sport Science Institute—particularly the brainwashing that has caused exercise enthusiasts and athletes to rush out and down electrolyte drinks, powders, and capsules during hot and humid exercise sessions. For nearly a decade, I was one of those athletes.

But here's the deal: your body is very, very good at regulating electrolyte status of the blood and cells. If it was not good at this, then you would die or become severely ill very easily if you were sweating without water intake for even a dozen minutes. And this just isn't the case.

Instead, when you have too little sodium on board, the body excretes less sodium in the kidneys, urine, and sweat, thus shutting down losses. And when you have too little water, the body excretes more sodium in the kidneys and sweat so that you maintain a proper electrochemical gradient.

Furthermore, when you have too much sodium, the body excretes excess sodium in the kidneys, urine, and sweat. And therein lies the rub: *people take a bunch of sports drinks or electrolytes to work out , find that they're losing lots of sweat or seeing white salt deposits on their skin, assume they're losing salt (oh no!) and begin a vicious cycle of consuming even more electrolytes.*

Noakes points out multiple studies that have shown people going for days with no salt or electrolyte intake and doing just fine at exercise. In one study, a group of soldiers performed an extremely intense march in the heat and humidity that lasted all day. Although they lost liters of sweat, all they did was drink water. No electrolytes. And at the end of the march, *their plasma sodium levels were the same as when they had started.* Their bodies simply held on to their salt stores. But studies like this get suppressed by sports drink manufacturers.

In addition, we're taught that the body has finite salt stores of about 10,000mg, so at normal salt losses of 1000-2000mg per hour, you could only go somewhere between 5 and 10 hours before you start to cramp. In reality, your salt stores are many, many times more than 10,000mg.

So if lack of electrolytes doesn't cause cramping, what does? In most cases, cramping is due to fascial adhesions and lack of mobility (revisit the mobility chapter), neuromuscular fatigue from pushing your muscles harder than you've pushed them in previous races or workouts, areas of scar tissue from previous injuries, or very low hydration levels. To learn more about this, listen to this Tri Talk Episode #74, which is an extremely thorough audio about mitigating muscle cramps.

Since I've spoken with Dr. Noakes, I've competed in over a dozen Half Ironman events, two Ironman triathlons, and multiple long training sessions in the heat with zero electrolytes, and did just fine, with zero cramping. The only people who may need to worry about electrolyte intake during exercise are folks who have been on a low-sodium or mineral-deficient diet for a long time, or people with medical conditions that can affect sodium retention and loss (such as hypothyroidism). So here's the deal: electrolytes aren't necessarily going to hurt you during exercise, but you should just know that there are probably better places to spend your supplement or exercise dollars than on useless capsules.

And water? It can all be summed up in one simple sentence: drink plain, clear water when you're thirsty. I highly recommend you by Dr. Tim Noakes and with him if you want to really delve into the detailed studies and science behind how much water to drink (and also how we've been lied to and misled by faulty research into both water and electrolytes).

Ultimately, the take-away message is that electrolytes aren't going to hurt you, but they're not as crucial as you think . . . and excessive water intake can definitely hurt you so you should simply drink when you're thirsty.

Experiment with any of this in training before you take it into something like a triathlon, ultrarun, or marathon. You'll be far more mentally confident if you do

A Sample Ironman Race Day Fueling Protocol

Let's finish by applying everything that you've just learned to a sample fueling protocol for one of the most nutritionally confusing events on the face of the planet: the Ironman triathlon (incidentally, you can simply take bits and pieces of this approach and use it for a Half Ironman, a marathon, etc.).

1. About two hours before the race, eat a meal of 600-900 calories. You'll need to experiment with the exact amount in training. If you're wanting to stay low carb prior to your race, this can be 12–16oz of Bulletproof Coffee, or 12–16oz Ketogenic Kale Shake, or 1–2 servings of UCAN SuperStarch in coconut milk. For higher carbohydrate intake, eat a couple baked sweet potatoes or yams with sea salt, or 2 cups of cooked white rice. In either scenario, mix into these meals 1–2 tablespoons of or coconut oil and for even more calories, 1–2 tablespoons of a cold-press plant-based oil such as Udo's Oil or Panaseeda Five Oil Blend. Also include 20–30 grams of a hydrolyzed whey protein (such as Mt. Capra's DEEP30 protein); 5–10 grams of essential amino acids or 10–20 grams of a hydrolyzed collagen protein source (such as Great Lakes or Bernard Jensen). Once you mix all this together, it will form a thick, gel-like texture in your water bottle.
2. Drink plain, clear water from breakfast up until the swim start, and if necessary, for an extra hit of energy prior to the swim, have one of the fat-based energy gels.
3. On the bike, mixed into a downtube water bottle, consume for each hour the following: 1–2 servings SuperStarch or ISKIATE, 1–2 tablespoons MCT oil, and 5–10 grams of essential amino acids. Optionally, you can include one serving of VESPA every two to three hours

on the bike. If you decide you're going to use electrolytes, also mix them into this same bottle (if using capsules instead of powder, you can break open capsules if necessary). You should ideally have one bottle of this fuel mixed for the first half of the bike ride already on your bike's downtube, then the other half waiting for you at the special needs station for the race. Be sure to mix, stir, or even blend your bottle's contents well and give it a good shake prior to each dosing, as dense mixtures like this tend to "clump." Drink plain water when you're thirsty, from a separate bottle.

4. On the run, you have a couple options. You can do exactly as you did on the bike, but instead of water bottles, you can use a running flask or fuel belt. I prefer the Nathan Sports Vapor Shot flask, which is very ergogenic and easy-to-hold. You can use one flask for the first half of the marathon and simply have another flask waiting for you in special needs for the second half of the marathon. Continue to drink water when thirsty, and optionally, continue to include one serving of VESPA every two to three hours (e.g,. in bike-to-run transition and in special needs for run). The other option is to simply eat a fat-based energy gel every 20–30 minutes (the larger you are and the faster you're moving, the more frequently you may find you need to eat one).
5. Cross the finish line with a smile on your face, free of gut rot and much lower on AGEs and ROSs than you would have been if you'd been stuffing your face with simple sugars for the past day.

What About When You Do Need to Eat Carbohydrates From Grains & Legumes?

As an athlete, and especially as an endurance athlete, it can be difficult sometimes to actually get all the carbohydrate that you need from just rice and potatoes. Not only can that lead to "food boredom," but it can sometimes be tough or inconvenient to find these foods when you're traveling to races or at restaurants.

So although "safer starches" like rice, sweet potatoes, yams, or even fruit in moderation are better choices when you need to load up on carbohydrates for a workout or race, here is what you should do if you do need to choose alternative forms of carbohydrate like grains or legumes.

1. Avoid wheat, soybeans, and peanuts. You can listen to my interview (http://bit.ly/1KmAxJa) with Dr. William Davis to learn more about why to avoid wheat, but of all the grains, wheat is the most likely to cause rapid spikes in blood sugar and some serious digestive and gastrointestinal damage that can lead to immune system and performance problems. Most whole grain, whole wheat, and "healthy" packaged starches use wheat as a primary ingredient, so be careful! In addition, compounds called phytic acids can bind to minerals and inhibit absorption of the compounds necessary for optimum performance. Soybeans are very high in phytates as are peanuts (although phytates in soy can be significantly reduced through fermentation, which is why fermented soy such as miso, natto, and tempeh is OK, while unfermented sources such as tofu, soymilk, or edamame are not).
2. Soak & Sprout. Legumes, grains, nuts, and seeds have developed a natural protection against consumption by animals. This protection, which includes elements like saponins and phytic acids, allows them to resist digestion or irritate an animal's digestive system so that the legume, grain, nut, or seed can bypass digestion and be

"deposited" to grow elsewhere. This is an unpleasant paradox, but humans are smarter than plants, and by soaking and sprouting we can cause germination, which disables these protective mechanisms in the legume, grain, nut, or seed. Even if you don't sprout these foods, which is the ideal way to go, you can still soak them. Here is a great, free tutorial on soaking beans, legumes, grains, nuts, and seeds: (http://bit.ly/1KiRZdh).

Here is another great, free tutorial that will show you exactly how to sprout—which will allow you to eat foods like quinoa, amaranth, millet, or even "safer" forms of wheat like Einkorn wheat berries without the digestive issues or risk: (http://bit.ly/1LdcbSQ).

By avoiding wheat, soybeans, and peanuts, and actively soaking and sprouting your beans, legumes, grains, nuts, and seeds, you open yourself up to being able to consume without gut damage a larger variety of carbohydrates for those times when you actually do need more carbohydrates, such as during a race week, or on the day of a very hard or long workout.

8 Supplements That Help You Perform Better on a Low-Carbohydrate Diet

If you've spent much time on my blog: (bengreenfieldfitness.com), you probably know I've written several articles and produced several podcasts about how to practically implement a low-carbohydrate or a ketogenic diet, including:

Is It Possible To Be Extremely Active and Eat a Low Carbohydrate Diet?	http://bit.ly/1LdcFsc
Can You Build Muscle On a Low Carbohydrate Diet?	http://bit.ly/1VYy7UW
Should You Eat Carbohydrates Before Exercise?	http://bit.ly/1ORDRvw
How I Ate a High Fat Diet, Pooped 8 Pounds, and Then Won a Sprint Triathlon.	http://bit.ly/1VYycbt
The Hidden Dangers of a Low Carbohydrate Diet	http://bit.ly/1Obk2SQ

10 Ways to Do a Low Carbohydrate Diet the Right Way	http://bit.ly/1f4vIkZ
How To Become A Fat Burning Machine: Part 1	http://bit.ly/1owwZKv
How To Become A Fat Burning Machine: Part 2	http://bit.ly/18kTAU4
5 Simple Steps To Turning Yourself Into A Fat Burning Machine	http://bit.ly/1G5vuc8

But the reality is that it can be very, very difficult and uncomfortable to switch to a low-carbohydrate or "ketogenic" diet if you don't have the help of a few supplements, especially if you're serious about performance in sports like triathlon, Crossfit, marathoning, and other high-energy depleting events.

So now I'm going to tell you about eight supplements that can help you perform better on a low-carbohydrate diet, along with a couple footnotes at the end that I think you'll find very interesting.

1. Sodium.

When you shift to a low-carbohydrate or a ketogenic diet, your body loses storage carbohydrate and also begins excreting sodium and water. When this happens, your blood pressure quickly drops, and much of the low energy that is attributed to "low blood sugar" when eating low carbohydrate is actually due to this low blood pressure.

Because of this, if you experience feelings of lightheadedness or sluggishness (especially during your workouts), you should include extra sodium in your diet. One strategy is to get 1–2g of extra sodium during the day by using vegetable or chicken bouillon cubes. I personally do fine by simply using two or three effervescent electrolyte tablets each day (I use the Hammer

Nutrition fizz, which you can get 15% discount on with code 80244) combined with liberal use of Aztec sea salt on my meals. If you find yourself getting dizzy frequently, you'll need to especially be sure to include extra sodium (close to 1g is good) about 30 minutes prior to your workout.

If you already get 3–4g of sodium per day in your diet, this is probably a moot point for you, but it's pretty rare that I find hard-charging athletes following a low-carb diet to be consuming adequate minerals and electrolytes purely from food sources.

Caveat: the extra sodium is not because Tim Noakes was wrong in my interview with him. You don't need extra electrolytes during your workout to keep your muscles from cramping. This is simply extra sodium to help you maintain adequate blood plasma volume and blood pressure.

2. Branched Chain Amino Acids.

In my podcast episode "Do Amino Acids Really Help You Exercise Or Are Nutrition Supplement Companies Just Pulling A Fast One On You," you learned about branched chain amino acids (BCAAs).

The BCAAs are unique from other amino acids because the enzymes responsible for their degradation are low in your tissues, so they appear rapidly in the bloodstream and expose your muscle to high concentrations–ultimately staving off muscle breakdown and stimulating muscle synthesis, even during exercise.

BCAA supplementation after exercise has been shown to cause faster recovery of muscle strength and, even more interesting, the ability to slow down muscle breakdown—even during intense training and "overreaching" (getting very close to overtraining).

When you supplement with BCAAs, they can decrease the blood indicators of muscle tissue damage after long periods of exercise, thus indicating reduced muscle damage, and they also help maintain higher blood levels of amino acids, which can make you feel happy even when you're suffering during exercise.

But most important, if you're on a low-carbohydrate diet, when taken prior to a fasted exercise session, BCAAs could improve your fat oxidation and utilization of stored fatty acids as a fuel.

Dosage for BCAAs would be leucine, isoleucine, and valine in a 3g:1.5g:1.5g ratio. I personally just use whole amino acids (see below), but they're spendier, so if you want to go with BCAAs, you could use any of these options: (http://amzn.to/1OcjuZm).

3. Whole Amino Acids

Whole amino acids offer you all the benefits of branched chain amino acids, and then some. Whole amino acids (also known as essential amino acids, or EAAs) were essentially (pun intended) summed up in an article I wrote previously about EAAs:

"If all 8 essential amino acids are present, muscle repair and recovery can start before you're even done with your workout–and when you're mentally stretched towards the end of a tough workout, game, or race, high blood levels of amino acids can allow the body and brain to continue to work hard instead of shutting down."

This is all the more true if you're in a carbohydrate-depleted state.

Anyway, protein quality is typically determined based on the EAA profile of any given protein, and generally, animal and dairy products contain the highest percentage of EAAs, resulting in greater protein synthesis and post-workout recovery than vegetarian protein-matched control.

But you don't have to take a steak (or your pea and rice protein powder blend) out with you on your workouts. Most of the clients I coach are now simply popping 5–10 amino acids capsules or a couple scoops of amino acids powder during their long workouts or races, and are getting extremely fast absorbing EAAs in the process. Essential or whole amino acids can be spendy but if you want the best of AAs, this would be the way to go, at a dosage of 10g before very long workouts, then 5–10g every hour.

4. Glutamine

Glutamine plays a role in muscle glycogen synthesis and whole-body carbohydrate storage. This was first observed in a study in the American Journal of Physiology that found that an infusion of glutamine promoted a resynthesis of muscle glycogen stores that wasn't observed in a control group infused with alanine plus glycine.

An oral dose of glutamine at about 8 grams can promote storage of muscle glycogen to levels similar to consuming straight glucose, which is especially useful when you don't have much glycogen (storage carbohydrate) to go around due to a low-carbohydrate diet.

Glutamine supplementation has also been shown to enhance glucose production during exercise. Once again, if you're carbohydrate restricted in your diet, this can be good news. There's also some evidence that supplementation with glutamine may be effective for preventing immune suppression from strenuous exercise.

To use glutamine properly, you'd just take 8g of regular old glutamine immediately after your workout (avoid the glutamine powders with artificial sweeteners and additives). I should emphasize that if you want the ultimate combination of amino acids, electrolytes, and glutamine all at once, then bone broth is for you. You can learn everything you need to know about bone broth here, and can simply rotate 1–2 cups per day into your routine (e.g., a cup of bone broth with lunch and another cup with dinner).

5. Taurine

In a study entitled "Potentiation of the Actions of Insulin by Taurine," the amino acid taurine was shown to have a carbohydrate sparing effect. Taurine may also amplify the effect of insulin, allowing for more efficient carbohydrate utilization.

Research on taurine- and caffeine-containing beverages has shown that during prolonged endurance exercise, decreased heart rate and decreased catecholamine (stress hormones) are observed compared to using caffeine alone. Based on this, many folks will slam a Red Bull energy drink during a tough, long event.

But I don't recommend Red Bull for a variety of reasons, including the presence of artificial sweeteners and high amounts of citric acid. Instead, you can just take 2g of a taurine capsule or powder, about 30–60 minutes prior to a tough or long exercise session in a relatively carbohydrate-depleted state.

6. Medium Chain Triglyceride Oil or Coconut Oil.

When you exercise while on a low-carbohydrate diet, you're going to be burning lots of fatty acids as a fuel, and the medium chain triglycerides (MCTs) that you'll find in medium chain triglyceride oil and coconut oil can be a tremendous asset for keeping your energy levels high.

The stuff is easy to use: just take 2–3 tablespoons of coconut oil or 1–2 tablespoons of medium chain triglyceride oil about 30–60 minutes before you head out for a workout session. You could repeat this dosage every 2–3 hours during something like a long bike ride.

7. Magnesium

Although a low-carbohydrate diet doesn't massively deplete magnesium in the same way that it does sodium, upon switching to a low-carb diet (especially when combined with intense exercise) many people experience nighttime leg cramping and more muscle discomfort during exercise, and this is likely due to low magnesium.

About 70% of people don't get anywhere near enough magnesium, and if you're leaching magnesium with a combination of sweating and a low-carbohydrate diet, you're almost guaranteed to have some muscle twitching issues. Considering that over 300 enzymes require magnesium as a co-factor to make them work properly, it's a smart move to add magnesium into a low-carbohydrate diet.

I personally simply use a multivitamin complex that includes adequate amounts of many minerals, including magnesium. Some people like to use about 300-500 milligrams of something called "Natural Calm Magnesium" before bed at night (this can assist with sleep too). I also use a large application of topical magnesium oil on each leg immediately after my workouts. Magnesium can attract water into the colon, so back off the total amount of magnesium you consume if you get very loose stool.

8. VESPA

In the book *Art & Science of Low Carbohydrate Performance*, Jeff Volek and Steve Phinney mention a supplement called VESPA.

VESPA is basically a naturally occurring amino acid compound that is extracted from wasps. The theory behind this supplement is that wasps rely upon this amino acid to be able to travel extremely far distances on relatively low amounts of carbohydrate fuel and a relatively large reliance upon stored body fat. While there's not a huge amount of scientific evidence or clinical research data on VESPA, there are plenty of anecdotes that it can give some benefit to people who are training in a low-carbohydrate or ketogenic state. For example, ultrarunner Tim Olsen just won the brutal Western States 100 Mile Running Race and said:

"*On race day, I use VESPA, which is an amino acid supplement, about every 2hrs and a 100 calorie gel pack about every hour. Being on a low-carb diet helps me to efficiently burn fat as my fuel. The few cal an hour I use allow me to run as fast as I can . . .*"

Summary

So let's say you want to get every advantage possible, you want to use supplements, you're gearing up for a killer exercise session, or a big event like a marathon or a triathlon, you're eating a low-carbohydrate diet, and you're not wanting to carbohydrate load or use lots of carbohydrate during your big workout or event. Based on what I've written in this chapter, here's what you do:

30–60 minutes prior: 1g sodium (e.g., a chicken bouillon cube) or 2–3 electrolyte tablets, 5–10g BCAAs or EAAs, 2–3 tablespoons medium chain triglyceride oil or coconut oil, 2g taurine, and a generous amount of topical magnesium on each limb.

Every hour during: 5–10g BCAAs or EAAs, and then optional, but recommended if you're moving hard for multiple hours + 1 serving VESPA + everything else you learned about for carb/fat/protein intake from the previous chapter.

Immediately after: 8g glutamine or a cup of bone broth.

Closing Thoughts

If you've made it this far, then you know more than 99% of the world's athletic population when it comes to fueling your body for the combination of ideal health and performance, and you're now completely prepared for metabolic efficiency, weight loss, longevity, and breaking the sugar addiction.

So now it's time for you to head out into the trenches and start implementing what you've learned. Visit the grocery store. Reboot your pantry and refrigerator. Make it through those first two "uncomfortable" weeks of fat adaptation. Go!

Finally, if you have questions about what you've read, then you have a few options.

For a one-time Q&A, just ask a question over on my free podcast. You can ask a question using the "Ask Ben" form on the right sidebar of the website, you can download the free iPhone or Android app and ask your question that way, or you can call 1-877-209-9439 and leave an audio question via the phone or Skype.

I also do personal consulting and one-on-one phone calls for more intensive Q&A or for conversations that are more detailed. I'd be happy to help you via one of these personal one-on-one consults. Just go here and then choose a 20 or 60-minute consult, whichever you'd prefer. I can schedule ASAP after you get that: (greenfieldfitnesssystems.com/product/ben-greenfield).

Ben Greenfield

P.S. One last thing: if you enjoyed this book or found it useful, I'd be incredibly grateful if you'd post a short review on Amazon. Your support really does make a difference, and I read all the reviews personally so I can get your feedback to make this book and future titles even better. If you'd like to leave a review, all you need to do is go here: (http://amzn.to/1EYTNfN).

Thanks again for your support!

Thank You!

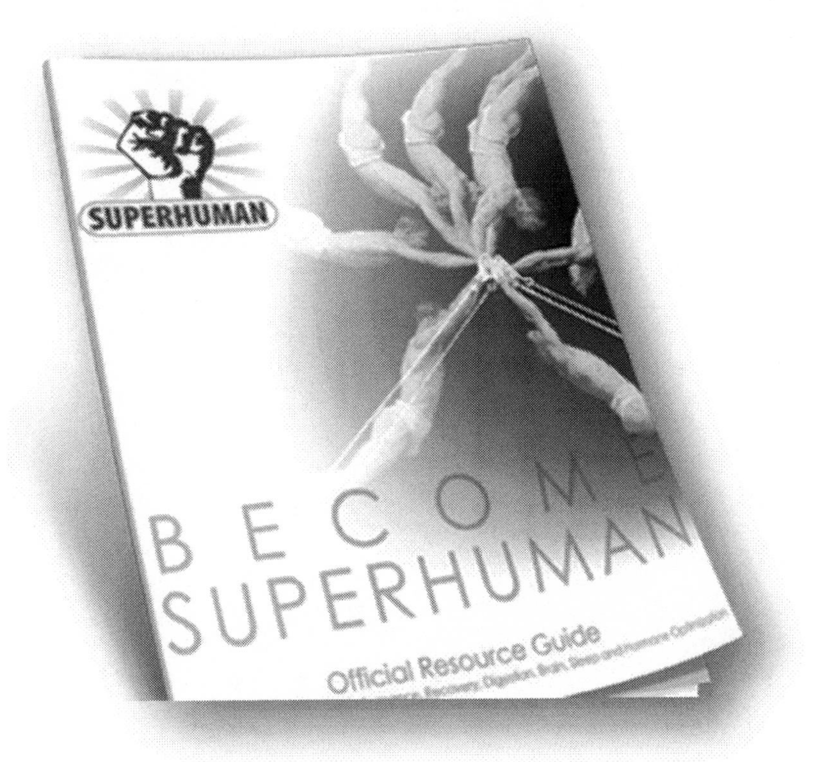

Thank you for taking the time to read this book. I'm now going to give you a FREE copy of my "Superhuman Resource Guide," discount coupons, a complete audio book summary of this entire book, and a secret bonus I prepared that I think you will really enjoy! Go here to grab your free low-carb book bonus now: (bengreenfieldfitness.com/low-carb-diet).

Other Books by Ben Greenfield

- *Get Fit Guy's "Secrets To A Better Workout"* **FREE!**
- *Get-Fit Guy's Guide to Achieving Your Ideal Body*
- *Become Superhuman: Official Resource Guide*
- *Weight Training For Triathlon: The Ultimate Guide*
- *Shape21: The Lean Body Manual*
- *Endurance Planet's Guide to Elevation*
- *The Low Carbohydrate Diet For Triathletes*
- *100 Ways To Boost Your Metabolism*
- *Holistic Fueling For Ironman Triathletes*
- *REV Diet*
- *Quick And Dirty Tips For Life After College*
- *Real Food Basics: Recipes For Your Long Workout*
- *How To Qualify For Kona*
- *Endurance Planet's Guide To Triathlon Spectating*
- *Personal Trainer's Guide To Earning Top Dollar*
- *Endurance Planet's Big Book Of Bravado*
- *Run With No Pain*
- *Endurance Sports For Kids*

References

PAGE 1

1. Rewriting the Fat Burning Textbook: Part 1 - http://www.bengreenfieldfitness.com/burnfat
2. Rewriting the Fat Burning Textbook: Part 2 - http://www.bengreenfieldfitness.com/burnfat2

PAGE 2

3. "How Much Carbohydrate, Protein and Fat You Need To Stay Lean, Stay Sexy and Perform Like a Beast." http://www.bengreenfieldfitness.com/carbprofat
4. organizations such as DNAFit - https://greenfieldfitnesssystems.com/product/dnafit/

PAGE 3

5. "Five Simple Steps To Turning Yourself Into a Fat Burning Machine." - http://www.bengreenfieldfitness.com/5steps
6. digestive enzymes - https://greenfieldfitnesssystems.com/hcl

PAGE 4

7. protein toxicity - http://www.bengreenfieldfitness.com/toxicity

PAGE 5

8. http://www.cholesterol-and-health.com/

PAGE 11

9. MCT - http://medical-dictionary.thefreedictionary.com/MCT
10. branched chain amino acids or essential amino acids - https://greenfieldfitnesssystems.com/aminos
11. medium chain triglyceride oil - https://greenfieldfitnesssystems.com/mctoil
12. coconut oil - https://greenfieldfitnesssystems.com/coconutoil
13. "Infinit-E" by Millennium Sports - http://www.millenniumsport.net/
14. "ISKIATE Endurance" by Natural Force - http://www.mynaturalforce.com/#bengreenfield

PAGE 12

15. read this helpful article about my own pantry. - http://www.bengreenfieldfitness.com/pantry
16. your specific needs and deficiencies - https://greenfieldfitnesssystems.com/product-category/lab-testing/
17. a high-quality multivitamin - http://www.bengreenfieldfitness.com/multi
18. daily electrolyte supplement - https://greenfieldfitnesssystems.com/product/catalyte-isotonic-lemon-lime-electrolytes/
19. fish oil - https://greenfieldfitnesssystems.com/fishoil
20. use 10% discount code BEN here - http://www.energybits.com/
21. a workout and injury recovery supplement that contains natural anti-inflammatories -

https://greenfieldfitnesssystems.com/product/naturefl ex-bone-and-joint-healing-supplement/

22. adaptogenic herb complex - https://greenfieldfitnesssystems.com/product/tianchi-chinese-adaptogenic-herb-complex/

PAGE 15

23. Thrive Market - http://bengreenfieldfitness.com/thrive

PAGE 16

24. USWellnessMeats - http://www.grasslandbeef.com/StoreFront.bok?affId=136074

PAGE 17

25. Bone Broth - http://greenfieldfitnesssystems.com/brothery

PAGE 18

26. Fuel SuperGreens - https://greenfieldfitnesssystems.com/supergreens
27. Living Fuel SuperProtein - https://greenfieldfitnesssystems.com/livingprotein

PAGE 20

28. a fan of this recipe - http://wellnessmama.com/223/turmeric-tea-recipe/
29. all coffee details/recipe here - http://www.bengreenfieldfitness.com/easymeals
30. This High Fat Smoothie - http://www.bengreenfieldfitness.com/smoothie

PAGE 21

31. sweet potato fries. - http://www.bengreenfieldfitness.com/sweetpotato
32. Spicy Shrimp & Onions. - http://www.bengreenfieldfitness.com/shrimp

PAGE 23

33. a big fan of these, click here - http://www.bengreenfieldfitness.com/pasta

PAGE 27

34. HERE - http://www.hammernutrition.com/
35. US Wellness Meats - http://goo.gl/Bllzc
36. all-natural jerky from US Wellness Meats. - http://goo.gl/Bllzc
37. Warrior bars from Onnit - https://www.onnit.com/?a_aid=bengreenfield
38. Living Fuel Supergreens - https://greenfieldfitnesssystems.com/supergreens
39. Superberry - https://greenfieldfitnesssystems.com/superberry
40. organic, BPA-free coconut milk - https://greenfieldfitnesssystems.com/cocomilk

PAGE 28 - 29

41. http://www.GreenfieldFitnessSystems.com
42. branched chain amino acids or essential amino acids - http://greenfieldfitnesssystems.com/aminos
43. fat-based energy gel of your choosing - http://www.bengreenfieldfitness.com/gel
44. NaturalForce - http://www.mynaturalforce.com/#bengreenfield

45. mushroom teas - http://store.foursigmafoods.com/#_1_23
46. glass of red wine - http://www.bengreenfieldfitness.com/wine

PAGE 33

47. LivingProtein - https://greenfieldfitnesssystems.com/livingprotein
48. Barefoot Provisions - http://barefootprovisions.com/#_a_cBG1

PAGE 36

49. http://www.GreenfieldFitnessSystems.com

PAGE 43 - 44

50. Use 10% discount code "BEN" - http://www.energybits.com/
51. good dark chocolate - https://greenfieldfitnesssystems.com/darkchoco
52. Aztecan sea salt - http://www.bengreenfieldfitness.com/seasalt
53. vegan protein - https://greenfieldfitnesssystems.com/livingprotein
54. vanilla powder - http://tinyurl.com/vanpow

PAGE 47

55. Aztecan sea salt - http://www.bengreenfieldfitness.com/seasalt

PAGE 48

56. GreenfieldFitnessSystems.com - http://www.greenfieldfitnesssystems.com/

57. this article on the best ingredients for energy bars - http://www.bengreenfieldfitness.com/bars

PAGE 50

58. Real Food Recipes For Your Long Workouts - https://greenfieldfitnesssystems.com/realfood

PAGE 52

59. bitter melon extract - https://greenfieldfitnesssystems.com/product/mpx100-fat-burner/
60. digestive enzymes - https://greenfieldfitnesssystems.com/digestiveenzyme
61. healthy dark" chocolate - https://greenfieldfitnesssystems.com/darkchoco
62. Part 1 - http://www.quickanddirtytips.com/getfitguy244
63. Part 2 - http://www.quickanddirtytips.com/getfitguy245

PAGE 55

64. Go here to read up on FODMAPs - http://tinyurl.com/fixgut

PAGE 57

65. this blog article, in which I talk about why these things are also a fast track to the average person getting fat. - http://tinyurl.com/how2getfat

PAGE 58

66. blender - http://pacificfit.net/items/omni-blender/
67. Vitamix - http://tinyurl.com/vitablender
68. Omega masticating juicer - http://tinyurl.com/ojuicer
69. Magic Bullet - http://tinyurl.com/mgcbullet

70. olive oil - https://www.freshpressedoliveoil.com/a/APSHN001_Q313/dl

PAGE 59

71. carbohydrate/fat/protein ratios recommended earlier - http://www.bengreenfieldfitness.com/carbprofat

PAGE 60

72. ketogenic diet - http://www.bengreenfieldfitness.com/ketodiet
73. This comes out to about 30 grams, or 120 calories of carbohydrate. - http://tinyurl.com/30calcarb
74. Bulletproof Coffee - http://www.gopjn.com/t/S0BMSEZFQEpDRUdDQERDQ0pGRQ
75. Ketogenic Kale Shake - http://tinyurl.com/ketoshake
76. UCAN SuperStarch - https://greenfieldfitnesssystems.com/ucantub
77. MCT oil - https://greenfieldfitnesssystems.com/mctoil
78. coconut manna - http://tinyurl.com/cocmanna
79. MCT - https://greenfieldfitnesssystems.com/mctoil
80. Udo's Oil - http://tinyurl.com/bgfudo
81. Panaseeda Five Oil Blend - http://tinyurl.com/5oilblend

PAGE 61

82. You can read about that story here. - http://www.activationproducts.com/jointventures?AFFID=126333
83. Mt. Capra's DEEP30 protein - https://greenfieldfitnesssystems.com/deep30

84. essential amino acids capsule or powder - https://greenfieldfitnesssystems.com/?s=aminos&post_type=product
85. Great Lakes - http://tinyurl.com/gr8lake
86. Bernard Jensen - http://tinyurl.com/bernjen

PAGE 62

87. SuperStarch, - https://greenfieldfitnesssystems.com/ucantub

PAGE 63

88. ISKIATE Endurance fuel, made by Natural Force - http://www.mynaturalforce.com/ - bengreenfield
89. Research shows - http://firefitsteeringgroup.co.uk/fatmetabolismathlete.pdf

PAGE 64

90. amino acid complex derived from the Asian Mandarin Vespa Wasp - https://greenfieldfitnesssystems.com/wasp
91. “Floe” bottle - http://www.bengreenfieldfitness.com/racediet

PAGE 65

92. You can click here to read an article I wrote in which you will find 12 fat-based alternatives to sickeningly sweet sugar-based sport gels. - . http://www.bengreenfieldfitness.com/gel

PAGE 66

93. Oxidation of Solid versus Liquid Carbohydrate Sources - http://www.ncbi.nlm.nih.gov/pubmed/20404762%E2%80%8E
94. along with lots of anecdotal evidence among professional cyclists - http://www.slowtwitch.com/Interview/Up_close_with_Allen_Lim_3054.html
95. Here's an interesting study on triathletes - http://www.ncbi.nlm.nih.gov/pubmed/7751072

PAGE 68

96. How You're Being Manipulated By The Sports Drink Industry And What You Can Do About It - http://www.bengreenfieldfitness.com/2012/06/waterlogged/

PAGE 69

97. mobility chapter - http://www.bengreenfieldfitness.com/2013/05/mobility-for-endurance-athletes/
98. extremely thorough audio about mitigating muscle cramps. - https://itunes.apple.com/us/podcast/tri-talk-triathlon-podcast/id177585541

PAGE 70

99. fat-based energy gels - http://www.bengreenfieldfitness.com/gel
100. VESPA - https://greenfieldfitnesssystems.com/wasp
101. Nathan Sports Vapor Shot flask - http://tinyurl.com/shtflsk

PAGE 72

102. listen to my interview with Dr. William Davis - http://www.bengreenfieldfitness.com/2011/12/the-shocking-truth-about-wheat/

PAGE 73

103. Here is a great, free tutorial - http://nourishedkitchen.com/soaking-grains-nuts-legumes/
104. Here is another great, free tutorial - http://www.thenourishinggourmet.com/2008/12/sprouting-grains-2.html

PAGE 75 - 76

105. my blog - http://www.bengreenfieldfitness.com
106. Is It Possible To Be Extremely Active and Eat a Low Carbohydrate Diet? - http://www.bengreenfieldfitness.com/lowcarbex
107. Can You Build Muscle On a Low Carbohydrate Diet? - http://www.bengreenfieldfitness.com/lowcarbbuild
108. Should You Eat Carbohydrates Before Exercise? - http://tinyurl.com/gfgcarb
109. How I Ate a High Fat Diet, Pooped 8 Pounds, and Then Won a Sprint Triathlon. - http://www.bengreenfieldfitness.com/squat
110. The Hidden Dangers of a Low Carbohydrate Diet - http://www.bengreenfieldfitness.com/lowcarbdanger
111. 10 Ways to Do a Low Carbohydrate Diet the Right Way - http://www.bengreenfieldfitness.com/10wayslowcarb

112. How To Become A Fat Burning Machine: Part 1 - http://www.bengreenfieldfitness.com/2014/05/how-much-fat-can-you-burn/
113. How To Become A Fat Burning Machine: Part 2 - http://www.bengreenfieldfitness.com/2014/05/how-much-fat-can-you-burn-2/
114. 5 Simple Steps To Turning Yourself Into A Fat Burning Machine - http://www.bengreenfieldfitness.com/2014/12/5-simple-steps-to-turning-yourself-into-a-fat-burning-machine/

PAGE 77

115. Hammer Nutrition - http://www.hammernutrition.com
116. Aztec sea salt - http://www.bengreenfieldfitness.com/seasalt
117. my interview with him - http://www.bengreenfieldfitness.com/2011/08/episode-157-the-death-of-gatorade-should-you-stop-using-electrolytes-during-exercise/
118. Do Amino Acids Really Help You Exercise Or Are Nutrition Supplement Companies Just Pulling A Fast One On You - http://www.bengreenfieldfitness.com/2011/04/do-amino-acids-really-help-you-exercise-or-are-nutrition-supplement-companies-pulling-a-fast-one-on-you-part-2/

PAGE 78 - 79

119. use any of these options - http://amzn.to/1OcjuZm
120. this article I wrote previously about EAAs - http://www.bengreenfieldfitness.com/2011/04/do-

amino-acids-really-help-you-exercise-or-are-nutrition-supplement-companies-pulling-a-fast-one-on-you-part-2/

121. 5–10 amino acids capsules or a couple scoops of amino acids powder - https://greenfieldfitnesssystems.com/?s=aminos&post_type=product
122. Glutamine - http://tinyurl.com/gltamne
123. Taurine - http://tinyurl.com/taurine12

PAGE 80 - 81

124. 70% of people don't get anywhere near enough magnesium - http://www.bengreenfieldfitness.com/running
125. multivitamin complex - http://www.bengreenfieldfitness.com/multi
126. Natural Calm Magnesium - https://greenfieldfitnesssystems.com/product/natural-calm-magnesium-powder/
127. topical magnesium - http://www.magneticclay.com/120-MagnesiumOil-72-custom.html

PAGE 81

128. Art & Science of Low Carbohydrate Performance - http://tinyurl.com/artscie
129. ultrarunner Tim Olsen just won the brutal Western States 100 Mile Running Race - http://tinyurl.com/timolsen

PAGE 82

130. EAAs- http://tinyurl.com/mapamino

PAGE 83 - 84

131. my free podcast. - my free podcast.
132. download the free iPhone or Android app - http://www.bengreenfieldfitness.com/app
133. Just click here - http://greenfieldfitnesssystems.com/product/ben-greenfield/
134. Beyond Training: Mastering Endurance, Health and Life - http://www.beyondtrainingbook.com/
135. BenGreenfieldFitness.com - http://www.bengreenfieldfitness.com/
136. all you need to do is click here - http://www.bengreenfieldfitness.com/ben-greenfield

PAGE 85

137. Ben's books - https://greenfieldfitnesssystems.com/product-category/books-programs/

PAGE 86

138. "Superhuman Resource Guide," - http://www.bengreenfieldfitness.com/low-carb-diet/
139. Click here to grab your free low-carb book bonus now. - http://www.bengreenfieldfitness.com/low-carb-diet/
140. "Superhuman Resource Guide," - http://www.bengreenfieldfitness.com/low-carb-diet/
141. Get Fit Guy's "Secrets To A Better Workout" - http://amzn.to/1eZs377
142. Get-Fit Guy's Guide to Achieving Your Ideal Body - http://amzn.to/1bzWKSz

143. Become Superhuman: Official Resource Guide - http://amzn.to/1jjacPM
144. Weight Training For Triathlon: The Ultimate Guide - http://amzn.to/1nY84NF
145. Shape21: The Lean Body Manual - http://amzn.to/1e7AHzl
146. Endurance Planet's Guide to Elevation - http://amzn.to/1aQxXWV
147. The Low Carbohydrate Diet For Triathletes - http://amzn.to/1bfvAAh
148. 100 Ways To Boost Your Metabolism - http://amzn.to/MvX7UN
149. Holistic Fueling For Ironman Triathletes - http://amzn.to/1du0yRX
150. REV Diet - http://amzn.to/1eCPre8
151. Quick And Dirty Tips For Life After College - http://amzn.to/1kiuSrd
152. Real Food Basics: Recipes For Your Long Workout - http://amzn.to/1g6S6zD
153. How To Qualify For Kona - http://amzn.to/1evRbYc
154. Endurance Planet's Guide To Triathlon Spectating - http://amzn.to/1fM42nZ
155. Personal Trainer's Guide To Earning Top Dollar - http://amzn.to/1b6G3k8
156. Endurance Planet's Big Book Of Bravado - http://amzn.to/1bzT1V5
157. Run With No Pain - http://amzn.to/1eBmwn7
158. Endurance Sports For Kids - http://amzn.to/1dTuNYs

About the Author

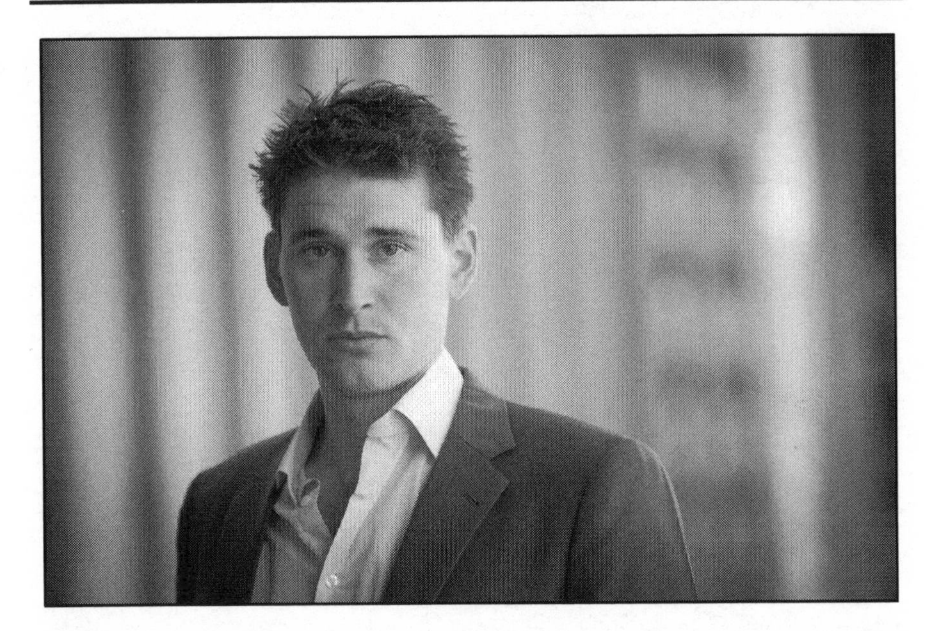

Ben Greenfield is an ex-bodybuilder, Ironman triathlete, Spartan racer, coach, speaker, and author of the New York Times Bestseller "Beyond Training: Mastering Endurance, Health and Life." In 2008, Ben was voted as NSCA's Personal Trainer of the Year and in 2013 and 2014 was named by Greatist as one of the top 100 Most Influential People in Health and Fitness. Ben blogs and podcasts at BenGreenfieldFitness.com and resides in Spokane, WA, with his wife and twin sons. To learn more details about Ben, go here: (bengreenfieldfitness.com/ben-greenfield).

You can find all of Ben's books by going here: (http://bit.ly/1QBevDy).

53253439R00068

Made in the USA
San Bernardino, CA
10 September 2017